WAS I NOT SUPPOSED TO SAY THAT?

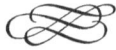

SARA SPRINGER

Copyright © 2024 Starfish Stories Publishing

Library and Archives Canada Cataloguing in Publications.

Copyright in Ontario Canada & Waco, Texas.

For permissions contact:

hello@starfishstoriespublishing.com

E-Book ISBN: 978-1-990419-35-5

Print ISBN: 978-1-990419-36-2

Hardcover ISBN: 978-1-990419-35-5

1st Edition

Edited by: C.B. Moore

Cover Designed by: Lauren da Silva

Photography by: Jennifer Hunn (Sweet as Hunny Photography)

For Words

For Lance, Aidan, Laila, Eli, Ava, and Amelia. Without you, I'd still be broken.

For you—yes you holding these words in your hands—I'm holding you in my heart. Keep going; I promise you'll be glad you did.

CONTENTS

PART II

Part II
FAIRY-TALE FODDER

PART III

Part III
BALANCE AND BULLSHIRT

PART IV

Part IV
LOVE LETTERS

IT GOES WITHOUT SAYING

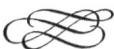

Oy vey. I am envisioning an epic introduction to the words of a book that will transform the lives of approximately no people, and I am already having second thoughts about putting said book into the world.

I want this memoir—of sorts—to be about overcoming mental illness. I mean *really* overcoming it. Like, kicking-its-rear-and-taking-its-name level overcoming. However, for this story to be honest I have to admit that I am a trauma survivor.

Pause for dramatic effect.

Well, since I am being honest, I am pausing to catch my breath because that, friends, is something I am not entirely ready to talk about but have accepted that I must. It is so deeply interwoven into every aspect of my life that I cannot try to cut it out and then piece this story back together without mentioning the vulture who took everything that made me feel whole and safe.

All right, so what trauma am I talking about?

Deep breaths, everyone...

I am a sexual abuse survivor. There. I said it. Because those words elicit a chest-tightening, heart-racing response as I type them out, I shall henceforth and forevermore refer to the abuse I experienced as the "Thing."

Now, I am not going to rehash the traumatic events. There are some writers who can share their pain delicately and beautifully. I am not that writer, nor am I that advocate. Still, there are a few details that should be mentioned about the Thing because those details shape my story, my faux healing, my breakdown, and my actual healing. Those details include the fact that it happened when I was eight—on more than one occasion—but I told no one until I was fourteen. The telling of the Thing was nearly as traumatizing as the Thing itself, so after the first telling I did not talk about it again until I was eighteen. And then again at twenty-three. And twenty-three was when I got serious about overcoming the Thing, mostly because I was pregnant with my first child and refused to burden him with a mother who was not sure she could keep herself breathing long enough for one more tomorrow.

I know my Thing is not as devastating as other things. If we were going to rate trauma—which, by the way, we should not—but for kicks and grins, if we were going to, I would say mine was middle-of-the-road awful. I personally know warriors who have survived much more horrific abuse than me. In fact, I often find myself asking: Was it really that bad? Am I overreacting? Did it really happen the way I remember it?

To be honest, I do not know the answers to any of those questions. All I know is that it broke me. It broke me in a way that the subsequent piecing-back-together-of-myself has been —and quite honestly, still is—fragile. So fragile that, much like a single rock can shatter a windshield without warning, so can one trigger shatter my sense of self into oblivion.

I have often wondered if I would have depression had I not

been rendered helpless and hopeless by my abuser. I do not have tangible evidence to support this theory, but I think it makes sense that all those years of silence shaped my brain, rewiring it in ways that the only emotions that could latch on to it were depression and anxiety. Unfortunately, in my experience this is a fairly common occurrence for survivors of abuse. I often wonder how much mental illness can be attributed to trauma over genetics. How many of us are hurt so deeply that there is no other outlet for our brains other than to cope by dissociating, shutting down, and becoming numb to our surroundings?

At one time I was given a statistic of the Thing happening to one in three people. That is an astoundingly large number. And yet we are afraid to discuss it and bring it to light. Not just we, but me.

I am afraid to talk about it. I do not want the *"You've got this"* and *"It'll be okay"* and *"I'm sorry that happened to you"* responses. I do not want people to see it when they see me. I spent a lot of years seeing myself as a villain incapable of stopping what should not have happened, and believing that because I could not stop it, I allowed it. Believing that because I allowed it, *I* was the monster. It is this type of misplaced blame that makes me grateful for therapy. In fact, it was during my very first session with my therapist of fifteen years that she said to me:

"Let us take this Thing and put it in a box. We acknowledge that it was awful and that it should not have happened. It was not your fault, and you did not allow it. We are not putting it away because we are forgetting about it. We are putting it into a box because it is only a piece of your past. It is not the whole story. So put it in that box. Now, tell me who you are."

That sound you are hearing? That is the sound of the wind

that was knocked out of me. For the first time in a long time, my mind drew a blank. Time stood still as I came to realize that my entire identity was wrapped around the Thing. I was a victim and nothing more. I must have drifted off into space for the remainder of my hour-long session because the next words I heard were:

"I want you to think about that over the next week. Come back to your next session and tell me who you are without that."

Oof.

Someone had finally said it. They had finally said something in response to my dirty little secret that was helpful and not hurtful. It was validating and liberating. Even so, the constant flashbacks kept piercing through my soul like shards of glass that refused to let old wounds heal. My brain was rewired—brainwashed, if you will—to believe that the antithesis of all she had said was true. I *was* the Thing. My regret was real. It gutted me over and over, even once I had surrendered to the guilt and begged it to leave me. It sensed my weakness and planted itself deeper into my psyche. As such, I think I came back that following session with a weakly formed response like: I am a friend, nurse, sister, daughter, wife and soon-to-be mother. I had no fucking clue who I was other than broken.

There you have it. That is my big secret. My big reveal. The assumed underlying contributor to my mental illness. The elephant in the room that is interwoven through this book.

I do not know where this fits into the moral of the story, but I feel unbelievably compelled to put these words in writing. If you ever find yourself at the receiving end of someone's confession that they were abused, I want to give you the tools to help them put that lousy piece of their story into a box. To help them ward off regret before it takes hold of their spirit and renders them hopeless.

Tell them that they did not do anything wrong.

Tell them that they did not deserve it.

Tell them that they could not have stopped it.

Tell them that it is not their shame to carry.

Tell them that they are not damaged or broken.

Tell them that they are worthy of being loved in healthy ways.

Tell them they matter, that it happened, and their pain is valid.

Tell them that the shame they feel is a liar and that by bringing it into the light, it will lose its power.

I have allowed shame to undermine me for long enough. It is time to heed my own advice and shine a big ol' light onto that shame. I am going to take away its power so I can reclaim my own. Maybe in the process, it will give you the strength to reclaim yours.

PART I

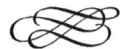

PART I
FINDING JOY

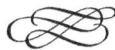

I have this idea to start each part with a "tie it all together" type paragraph or two, but I do not think this section really needs it. The title says it all. This is the story of how trauma had me in its death grip and how I found the light. It is also interspersed with tales of learning to accept my body, embrace my diversity, and advocate for those who have been suffering in silence.

It is also a reminder that mental illness is not something we conquer. It is something we cope with. It ebbs and flows. It is a journey. You will have good days and you will have bad days. Sometimes the bad days will outnumber the good ones, and sometimes they will linger for far too long.

But, trust me, the good days always come back around.

This is a story to encourage you to keep going. Even when it seems impossible. Even when the pain rises so high into your chest that you cannot breathe. Especially then.

Keep going. I promise you will find your joy.

UGH

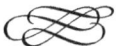

W ant to know what anxiety feels like?
It feels like death.

Heart exploding, cannot catch your breath, the weight of
your chest suffocating you. Begging with your eyes for
someone to help but not wanting to say anything because you
know they are tired of hearing it. I would be.

How many times can one person listen to another gripe
that they just cannot control their mind? They have therapists
for that; but alas a fifteen-minute appointment is not quite the
cure for daily doses of anxiety-provoking thoughts.

They have medication for that, but it is not always enough
to mute an overactive mind.

They have counselors for that, but you have to find the
strength to implement all the handy coping mechanisms you
learn. You also have to find the courage to say the words "I need
help" out loud.

Anxiety will hit me when I least expect it. I will first notice
it because any sound, from our dog barking to one of my chil-

dren softly saying "Mom" is deafening. Suddenly I am defensive and wondering why it is so loud. Why can I not just get a moment's peace? I am not always thinking when it happens, but my body tells me that I am overstimulated. I may as well have my head in a plastic bag because I am suffocating. I want to lie down in bed with a locked door and just sleep it off.

It hits me in the form of a midnight awakening turned into insomnia. Unable to sleep, arguing with my thoughts to be still and quiet. Spoiler alert: they do not listen.

It feels as though my brain wires are set on a default path of dramatization, overthinking, and catastrophizing pretty much any real or imagined scenario that pops in for a late-night rendezvous.

I have spent years trying to rewire my brain. Its default setting is still worrying. It takes work to redirect the flow of inner dialogue. First you have to recognize what is happening. It is hard when it seems rational. I am not worrying; I am simply preparing myself for any and all scenarios. I am learning not to spend emotional energy on things that have yet to happen. It is a process, one that does not come easily or naturally. In the past I coped with obsessive thoughts through distraction. That worked... for a while.

Actually, it did not work at all. Probably because I was not intentional in my distraction. I forced myself to ignore my thoughts. I have since learned to acknowledge them and let them go. Thoughts do not define you; they also are not fortune tellers predicting what we will be experiencing in the near to distant future.

They are just thoughts. Firings of a weary brain that picked up on something and decided to share it with my consciousness, which decided that I must have the incessant need to rip my skin from my bones and release all such thoughts and fears.

If you are wondering, yes, I am still talking about anxiety, and it is a demon in its own right. It is a painful knot in my stomach. It is nausea. It is my heart racing. My chest. I cannot take a deep breath in. I cannot breathe. I cannot breathe. It is so tight. I cannot breathe. It is overwhelm. I do not know what to do. Somehow, I get my bearings to open the door and try again.

Except one time.

I could not.

My kids ask a question.

"WHAT?" I snap.

Everything feels too much. Everything is too loud. I cannot breathe.

The tears well up in the corner of my eyes.

I excuse myself.

I lock myself in the bathroom. Doubled over with abdominal pain. Head in the toilet, sure as molasses that my guts will be coming out my mouth.

My skin is crawling. I need to rip it off. God, I wish I could. And then I cry. And cry. And cry.

Stop.

It is okay.

You can breathe.

Slow down.

Smell the roses, blow out the candles.

You can do this.

I call my husband.

"I think I need to go to the hospital."

"I'm coming home."

My nine-year-old son kneels down next to me and rubs my back.

"It will be okay, Mom."

13

Shit.

"Yes, it will. Thanks, bud."

My firstborn trying to talk me out of a panic attack.

I need help.

I called a physician-referral line the next day.

It took three phone calls to three different practices to find one doctor accepting new patients. And then it took two months for the first available appointment.

I just needed to make it to October.

...

I walk in.

"Have a seat."

Who would have thought that choosing a seat in a therapist's office would unleash such anxiety-ridden inner dialogue?

Does it matter which one I pick?

Does it mean something if I sit in the chair farther from him?

Or the one closest to the door?

Oh, just sit down, Sara.

"How are you doing?"

"Um, I'm fine."

I try to sound positive, but then I figure if I cannot be honest in a psychiatrist's office, then I am truly in trouble.

"What brings you here?"

"Anxiety and depression."

He asks a slew of questions. Takes down a history. A list of the anti-depressants I have tried and which failed, along with my current medications.

I am acutely aware of my movements.

A flurry of thoughts.

Stop moving your hands.

Stop bouncing your leg.

Am I making enough eye contact?

Am I making too much eye contact?

Does he think these movements are all made up?

... wait, are they?

"How are you tolerating Prozac?"

"I think it's helping. Definitely better than Zoloft and Paxil." I sound like a mess.

"Okay. Any nightmares?"

"Um, yea. Like graphic ones. For weeks on end. And then they will go away for a time and then come back. They really bother me."

"Any panic attacks?"

"Uh, all the time. My nine-year-old was there for my last one."

He makes a scrunched-up face.

"Ooph."

He pauses; seemingly to think.

"Well, sometimes Prozac can make anxiety worse, but since you seem to be tolerating it, I would like to increase your dose. And I would like to give you a low-dose beta blocker that will help alleviate some of these physical symptoms of your anxiety. But it can make you lightheaded. And something for sleep. To help with the nightmares. You are very symptomatic."

I am feeling oddly validated and surprisingly hopeful.

He hands me a prescription and says,

"Come back in two months and let's see how you are doing."

...

"How are you doing?"

"I think better."

"Good. Any nightmares?"

"I really don't think so."

"Good. Any panic attacks?"

"I think I have had like two or three this month. But I just do not feel like dealing with them; I pretty much can feel one coming on, so I take a Xanax. Is that wrong?"

"No, not wrong. So. Still having panic attacks?"

"Yea, but a lot less. I mean, before Prozac I was having them regularly."

I feel slightly defensive.

I am better.

I know I am.

Great, this is where he is going to tell me that he has done all he can and it is time to go back to the counselor which would be great except I have zero time to go to a counselor that would mean more time off work which is less on the paycheck and more bills not to mention all the gas it takes to get to her office or if I make an appointment for when I am off work then I have to find a babysitter which means I am paying for both a sitter and an appointment but if I just have someone come over for a couple hours it won't be that expensive.

Spiraling, exhausting thoughts interrupted.

"I think we should go up on the Prozac."

Taken aback.

"Really?"

"Yes, we are almost there—but you are still having symptoms, so I would like to increase the Prozac."

What does that mean?

"Wait. Are you telling me that it is possible for me to stop having panic attacks?"

"I think that is possible."

I am rendered speechless as I let that sink in.

"I didn't know what to expect. I didn't know what a realistic goal with medication was; like, what it was capable of and what I would have to keep dealing with."

"We are almost there."

Oddly validated and surprisingly hopeful.

LIGHT BRIGHT

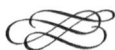

I have worked with counselors for approximately twenty-one years and with psychiatrists for the better part of four years. While I have made what I like to consider incredible progress over the years, there are still times I do not trust my own thoughts. Truly, I do not know when I am supposed to be afraid or worried or protective because I am always afraid, worried, and protective.

However, if my journey has taught me anything it is that the line between living with depression—or mental illness, for that matter—and dying by suicide is such a fine one that they are difficult to distinguish from one another. Being unable to believe your own mind and trust your own instincts is nothing short of a constant, exhausting brain teaser. The only thing that makes the tease less teasey is when we can get out of our own heads long enough to ask for help.

When inner demons are brought to light, they lose their power. I wish I could say that I came up with that fantastic line on my own, but no, I spent thousands of dollars in therapy learning that demons survive and thrive in the darkness.

I am going to drive that point home by inserting the word suicide.

Now I am going to ask you to pause.

What emotion does reading that word elicit? What objections to that word surface? What visceral reaction does your gut try to make you avoid?

And that is why we do not talk about it. It is uncomfortably uncomfortable.

But here is the thing, not talking about it is not helping anyone. Depression and anxiety should not be coined as invisible illnesses because, to those suffering, the pain is palpable. It must be acknowledged with the recognition that the consequences of untreated mental illness are literally devastating.

All that to say: even if it is unsettling to address and you feel like it's not okay and everything's pointless and you are stuck in such darkness and it's too overwhelming to even know where to start and you don't think you are strong enough to peel the layers because there is no healing and people make you feel like you are crazy or weak and that you don't have it that bad anyway or your battle is not legitimate because it's invisible, ask for help anyway.

Because even if it seems like it, you are not alone.

And even if it does not seem like it, you matter.

And even if it does not feel like it, you will get better.

And even if it does not feel like it, there is hope.

SNIPPETS AND SNAPSHOTS

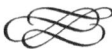

All of us have scattered memories of childhood. Bits and pieces that are not quite the full story but enough to start molding our values as we develop into adults. This chapter is kind of like video clips of home movies. I liken it to the scene in my go-to Christmas movie: *National Lampoon's Christmas Vacation.* There is a moment when Clark Griswold goes up into his attic to hide his family's presents, and in true *Vacation* fashion, he gets locked up there for several hours while his family is out enjoying a spirited afternoon of holiday shopping and lunch. While he is there, he discovers a box full of old home movies. The kind that is made of actual film and played on a projector. In these movies there are flashes from different moments of his life, enough to get the emotion of what was happening without really knowing the story behind it. A snippet—if you will.

Here are my snippets.

Once upon a time, I was born. I lived for a few years, and I do not remember much until I was three; that is my first memory. Most likely because I was lost on a beach.

Let us chat about that.

I remember flying a kite with my dad and asking him if I could go back with my mom. He said,

"Sure."

I am sure it seemed simple enough because, if you ask them, my mom was directly behind me, only a few feet away.

However, I believe that to be a big fat lie. I ran the entire length of that beach and never once saw her. Never mind everything looks the same to a three-year-old. I remember running and seeing a bunch of chairs and people in swimsuits and umbrellas. And then there were not any. I pulled a *Forrest Gump* and just kept running.

I vividly remember being afraid sharks would come to the shore to eat me. Weird I would have that fear when I do not remember when I would have been taught that sharks exist and that they will eat people.

I digress.

Next, I knew a man and woman driving a *Jeep*-like vehicle came up to me and said,

"Are you Sara Kur-ah-bet?"

"Yeah," I replied.

Apparently, the lesson to not talk to strangers never really sank in; I hopped right onto the nice lady's lap and she took me back to my parents since I have lived the rest of my early years with them raising me.

Glad that turned out well.

Fast forward three years. Kindergarten-aged. I just wanted to play house with friends on the playground.

"I am going to be the mom," says the ringleader.

She then points to another little girl and assigns her the role of her daughter.

Then my turn. *"And you will be the maid... because you have dark skin."*

In that moment I realized that my different look was noticeable, and that lighter tones were more appealing to others. That was the first time I remember being treated differently because of how I looked—and I can honestly say it was not the last.

I guess this would be as good a time as any to mention my physical features. I am your average five foot one and a half inches—that half has mattered most of my adult life. I am short and stocky with a girl-down-the-street vibe; I have never been popular enough to be the girl next door. I have coffee-with-creamer-colored eyes, even darker hair with sandy, olive skin tones. I do have a nose that can speak for itself. I have been told on more than one occasion, as a child and as an adult, that my nose is too big and that I must be Jewish. I have always found ignorance to be astounding, but I guess my nose has character.

I am an American citizen born and raised in the United States; more specifically, middle America. I was born to an American mother and Kuwaiti father. If you are thinking that sounds like an odd couple, you would be wrong. I spent my childhood idolizing their relationship. My dad always made my mom laugh harder than anyone else. I loved hearing her laugh. I would watch them hold hands in car rides and think, *"That's what I want."*

I always felt the only differences between them were their place of birth and religious preferences. Their divorce decades later proved me wrong.

I am a crossbreed between a Christian mother and Muslim father. These differences never seemed to hold any significance until they did, and the contradiction in their beliefs became a

23

pivotal component of my twisted confusion and my battles in this life.

Apparently, the way they spoke was also dissimilar. Over the course of my childhood, on more than one occasion I had friends who would politely remark:

"Your dad talks funny."

"How?"

"He says 'B' for everything."

Does he? I'd never noticed. Then I started listening.

"Bay-ber. Ben. Bibsi"

Translation: Paper. Pen. Pepsi.

I guess he does.

"Dad, why do you say bay-ber instead of paper?"

"In Arabic, there is only 'b' dah-lin."

"What's Arabic?"

"The language they speak in Kuwait."

"What's Kuwait?"

"It is where I was born."

"Can we go there?"

"One day."

I am sure that day came sooner and under more tragic circumstances than he had ever hoped for or expected.

Enter my next memory.

I remember him standing at the wet bar in the basement of our two-story home, frantically dialing a portable handset telephone.

I heard a broken voice coming through the speaker phone on the other side. He was talking in another language. One I was not familiar with. I had no idea what my dad was saying, but I could tell by his body language that something was wrong.

Iraq had invaded Kuwait.

I remember my dad being glued to the television on a daily basis, making desperate phone calls overseas to contact his family, trying to gather any information he could. His gaze seldom broke away from the television, and he would ask me on more than one occasion to bring him a fudgsicle. Who knows why my memory has held on dearly to that.

To my best recollection, he stayed holed up in the basement office, trying to obtain any information available about the unfolding situation.

Then the campaign *Free Kuwait* started.

His office space was filled with boxes of red t-shirts, and in big white letters they read:

"**FREE KUWAIT.**" Some with black lettering: "Students for a **FREE KUWAIT.**"

I still have one. It smells the same: old, musky, familiar.

Stickers pleading for a "**FREE KUWAIT.**"

He spoke to my first-grade class about it.

He gave interviews on television and radio about it.

I did not feel safe.

I remember having nightmares of Saddam Hussein coming into my classroom and taking me away. Geography does not play a role in a seven-year-old's fears. I remember the talk of threats to our family relating to my dad's campaigns and what that meant for our safety.

I remember seeing people on our lawn. They had video cameras. My mom would rush us past them into the car so our faces would not spend time on screen. I remember the mention of people calling and threatening our family. I did not understand because my dad was just trying to help.

I remember word that his brother, my uncle, had been

taken as a prisoner of war by Saddam Hussein making his way across the ocean to us. The effect that it had on him was heartbreaking and, truthfully, it still is.

We had family members fleeing into Saudi Arabia. My dad left the States to be with them; he was gone for six months. Unfortunately, as the years passed, his moving across the world for months or years at a time became a part of his identity. I think we have spent more time apart than together in my thirty-nine years.

Anyway.

Liberation came February 26, 1992.

Because America.

Next memory. My mom was sitting upstairs in the master bedroom, on her bed, talking to my dad on the phone.

"It's been six months."

I do not know what happened on the other end of that line, but apparently, we were moving.

Eight months after the liberation of Kuwait, we moved there. I remember descending into the country from above and seeing fires.

"The oil rigs are still on fire from the war," I remember my dad telling me as we stared out the window while landing in a war-torn country. We arrived at an apartment my grandfather had prepared for us. My dad provided my mom with a map.

"You are here, and here is everything else," he pointed out to her, in a nutshell.

I remember loving life there. Most of the kids at my school were like me: an American parent and a Middle Eastern parent; all of us with darker complexion, hair and eyes. Acceptance and fitting in. How important that is for a child.

We spent many a weekend at our family's beach houses. I loved every moment. We spent time fishing, playing unlimited rounds of card games like Uno and Spoon, and searching for seashells along the beachfront.

"Wah-wah-weese-weese."

That was the song we would sing for crabs to emerge from those shells. A catchy, rhythmic tune in a quiet tone always seemed the way to those crabs' hearts; they would emerge from their shells.

I was told on more than one occasion while seashell hunting, *"Do not pick up anything."*

After all, it could be a remnant of war. Shrapnel that could either detonate or be sharp enough to cause harm. It was a country trying to rebuild from devastation. I still think twice before picking up anything I come across, even as simple as a pen or coin.

I remember several occasions where Saddam Hussein was on the border threatening to invade. I remember the conversations between my parents about whether or not the threat was real; if we should stay or go.

There would be discussion and, at times, yelling.

"We are not staying here," I would hear my mom scream.

"You are safe, there is nothing to be worried about."

I always sensed my dad trying to reassure her. I remember one instance in particular.

"Sadam Hussein is on the border." She remained unconvinced that we were safe.

"There are American troops on the border! He is not coming in." His tone confident, it seemed like my dad wanted to laugh.

The love for America in this small country was endless.

They'd freed Kuwait. The certainty that radiated from my dad at having American troops on the border was reassuring; it has given me the utmost respect for the United States Armed Forces.

"We need to go to the American Embassy. We are going with or without you." She had decided.

No, this is not happening. At that moment, I entered their room crying.

The fighting stopped.

"I don't want to go with just you or you," I said sobbing as I pointed to each of my parents. *"I want to live with both of you."*

They motioned for me to come to them and hugged me.

"You aren't going anywhere. We are staying here," my mom said lovingly.

I remember being amazed that my mere presence and remarks were enough to change her mind. I remember hoping that we were really going to be safe. If we were not, then it would be my fault for asking them to stay.

That was the first time I remember wondering if my family was going to fall apart, and whether or not my fears of Sadam Hussein taking me away would materialize. I

never experienced war firsthand, but the threat of it has always seemed real.

Fear of invasion aside, I would not change living in my dad's homeland for anything. Well, except for one thing. This is where the Thing happened, and I would love to scrap that from my mind and act as if my time in a foreign country was nothing but an awe-inspiring experience of cultural diversity.

But I have lived that version of my story, and it did not get me very far.

I am not here to talk about what went down during those unpleasant moments. That is not my story. For starters, I am nowhere near strong enough to rehash those events and then go about my day as if it never happened. Reliving it is where the re-traumatization dwells, and I am just not a fan. Secondly, who really wants to read the words? I know I avoid all novels, stories, movies, and any form of expression where details of another's experience are discussed. Talk about a trigger warning.

However, I cannot ignore the fact that it has haunted me my entire life. These events are what led to my suicidal intentions and, therefore, they carry weight. I will simply say, it happened—and then all pure joy, contentment, and sense of safety left my spirit and were replaced with fear, confusion, and unbearable pain.

PH-ANTASTIC PHANTOMS

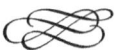

I never knew what was missing.
Or that it mattered that I missed it.
Or that it was a thing to miss.

Maybe I should start with what I am talking about, but I am afraid that once I say the words most of you will just close this book, no judgment, because this concept, in a way, is now saturating our social media feeds. But that does not make it any less important, poignant, or pertinent to those of us used to being under-represented in the media.

Oh, whoops. I said it. That is the writer's equivalent to a nip slip. I am talking about representation and how—nay, why —it matters. I mean, Netflix has this whole line of *Representation Matters* movies and shows, so obviously this is something worthy of discussion.

As I've mentioned, I am the exact antithesis of everything I always saw on television and movies growing up. Apart from my darker skin, I have crazy and coarse hair, especially if I do not use the right products—which I am still trying to find, by the way. I am not sure if my hair is curly or straight; it largely depends on the weather and my hormonal cycle.

I have bushy and coarse brows; I had no idea that soft brows existed. My eyebrows are like wires; literally, they feel like the string you use to go fishing.

I did not know what it was that I liked about living in Kuwait until I came back to the United States at thirteen and once again became the odd duck, on top of being an awkward teen. There was the nose which others felt the need to say made me look like a Jewish boy, and that was just one snap judgment my physical appearance inspired. For the record, I was convinced I would undergo rhinoplasty before I turned twenty, but somewhere along the line, I embraced the schnozz and now actually like it.

I was also the girl with dark upper lip hair that had to be bleached in secrecy before I graduated middle school, and heaven forbid anyone ever.

Find.

That.

Out.

Honestly, I thought that was a secret I would take to the grave. Thank goodness dermaplaning has become a fad we talk openly about. No more white cream burning into my upper lip while I wait the excruciating fifteen minutes for good measure to disguise the hairs the Good Lord gave me, only to find that six or seven stubborn hairs refused to conform, so bring out the tweezers to remove those bad boys.

Needless to say, I was not popular with the boys, despite my mother's insistence that "boys would be knocking down our doors." They, in fact, did not.

The shows I watched confirmed that what I looked like was not desirable. Often the person with a darker complexion was somehow a villain in whatever story was being told. The princes always seemed to fall for light-skinned and light-haired princesses. Disclaimer: I am not saying that is a bad thing; I am just saying that was how it seemed.

Magazines always seemed to have the delicate beauties on their covers. Tiny, under sloped noses with perfectly sun-kissed hairs and ocean-like eyes. Tiny chests and tiny waists with flat stomachs. All the things that my body fought against becoming.

To be honest, it wasn't until I was thirty-six that I realized how incredible it would have been to find myself represented in the world and in movies.

Enter *Julie and the Phantoms.*

One sleepless night, my kids asked to turn on Netflix, and we all snuggled up and started scrolling through our options. The beaded jacket on the cover of the title caught their attention, and against my better desires I agreed to turn it on. They fell asleep after two episodes, and I stayed up until 3 a.m. binge-watching a show that had me riveted.

Not only is it fun. Not only is it incredible. Not only can I sing along with the music. Not only am I blown away by the talent. But the main character reminded me of how I looked as a child.

She has the most beautiful black, corkscrew hair I have ever seen. Her complexion is perfectly olive.

Not to mention, her dad has an accent. Like mine did.

There is also a gay character. And that is just part of the story.

And they are all talented. And successful. And celebrated.

Not to mention, my tween self is thrilled at the fact that the "villain" in the story is a blond-haired light-skinned darling. Is that an immature response? Yes. Yes, it is. But apparently I have

33

a lot of pent-up aggression that I am just now recognizing and processing, so work with me.

The point of this whole story is that I think we undermine and undervalue the importance of being different. Sure, we say we celebrate differences and diversity matters and all that nonsense. But when we really look at what is put out into the world, does it reflect those supposed values?

I have seen plenty of the token-different-person; you know, the one who looks different than the rest but who is thrown in for comic relief or killed off pretty early on in the series or whatnot.

But true representation... where the main characters are still telling the same story... that is what has been missing.

These main characters and their stories and their physical appearance and their different backgrounds are refreshing and validating and inspiring and encouraging, and I just hope the trend continues because kids deserve to know that they are capable of the big things, regardless of their physical appearance and cultural background.

Not only are they capable, but they are also centerstage-worthy.

LONG STORY SHORT

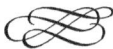

Believe it or not, the point of this story is not about planning a pity party or fishing for reassurance. The point of this story is twofold.

First off, I want to provide those who do not battle mental illness with insight as to what it is like to be affected by it. Odds are you know someone with anxiety or depression, or both, or another brain chemical imbalance that threatens to bring them to their knees. It is really hard to empathize with something you do not understand. It is even harder to support someone when the typical well-meant comments like "think positive" or "mind over matter" are moot. I think it is important to not only give those who battle the diseases the tools to fight, but to armor their support system—because, honestly, this internal war cannot be won in the depths of darkness and solitude.

Second, I want to tell all the warriors who have found themselves in the throes of intrusive thoughts that you are not alone. Not only are you not alone, but your story also deserves to be told. Your shame can survive in the light, and rather than just telling you that those two things are true, I am going to show you how those two things are true. These next few chapters expose my darkness in a way that is likely to make you uncomfortable, but it will also show how you can truly travel through the deepest darkness with your demons on your back and find your way to authentic joy and a light bright enough to keep you going.

Now, the reason for this almost-chapter is that there is a third group I worry about when reading the following pages: the group that is suffering or has suffered and will get triggered by what I am describing. I have been there—reading a book that promises inspiration and flashes me back to the Thing—and to be honest, I have not yet made my way through said books. I leave them tucked away at the bottom of my nightstand to avoid ever getting triggered again. To be honest, I wished they had a trigger warning so I could reap the benefits without succumbing to flashback, therefore I vowed to include trigger warnings when applicable in my story.

If you do not find inspiration or empathy in the details of someone's battles, honor that truth and skip ahead to Chapter 10: Semicolons and Circles.

That is when the light returns.

Just so you will not have any FOMO about it, I will fill you in on what the pages in-between say:

The Thing led me to depression.

Depression led me to guilt.

Guilt led me to hopelessness.

Hopelessness led me to darkness.

Darkness led me to suicidal ideation.

Suicidal ideation led me to treatment.

Treatment led me to healing.

And healing led me to truly living.

If you are skipping ahead to Chapter 10, I want to leave

you with this: you deserve to live life sans shame and accompanied by light. Not only do you deserve it, you can have it. You are not a damaged burden that needs to dissolve into the abyss.

Your brokenness is what makes you human.

Your resolve is what makes you brave.

Your faith is what makes you capable.

You, my friend, are a freaking warrior.

THINGS HAPPEN

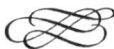

All right, I guess we are now at the part of the story where the Thing has happened, and as I alluded to previously, it happened while I lived in Kuwait. I am not rehashing any details, only saying that this is the part of the story where the hurt hits the fan.

I do not really know how to explain what happened after the Thing, but I think I faded into a shell of myself. I became hollow and empty, terrified, and ashamed. The guilt was unbearable; the loneliness was palpable. There is a level of awful that all of us probably have to go through to shape our resolve and find resistance, strength, and gratitude.

But trauma... that does not have to happen, does it?

The years of hiding and begging God to allow me to forget did shape me. One could argue that without them, I would never have become so passionate about helping others find mental health care, but there is a part of me that will not accept that something good came from the Thing.

My counselor recently asked me during a session to discuss my strengths; what I already like about myself. That caught me off guard. I can rattle off my weaknesses like nobody's business, but not so much anything positive. I had to dig deep to find the generic: "I guess I'm nice, and maybe sometimes kind of funny, and I think I can write." Committing to positives about myself has never been my strong suit, yet I thought maybe I nailed that one.

She disagreed and gave me an assignment to come back to my next session with actual examples of the good I have inside of me. That was a nearly unbearable ask, but I am nothing if not a rule-following assignment completer, so I did as asked.

I am sure you have heard it before that your trauma is not your fault, but your healing is your responsibility. I have always had an issue with that sentiment because healing is hard. It is a choice you have to make over and over and over again. It is so much easier to fall into the abyss of darkness and drown in the pain.

God, it is so much easier.

But darkness is heavy, and we can only carry the weight of our shame for so long before it will break us. When we are on the verge of brokenness, we have a choice: fall apart or put ourselves back together.

So, I will not give my abuser any credit for what I have overcome or for any "good" that my existence brings. Trauma may have made me desperate enough to find reasons for the suffering, but my ability to do so was earned by me and the ones who loved me through it all.

In case you are wondering, that is what I told my counselor at my following session.

FAKING HAPPY

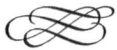

"*You are not the only one who has been through stuff.*"

That sentence has been uttered to me on many occasions throughout the decades of my life. It used to be nails on a chalkboard. I would react rather viciously and spew out,

"*You don't know what I've been through!*"

I have learned that they were right.

To be honest, my story is not that extraordinary. In fact, it is probably quite ordinary.

And that is why I have to tell it.

Let us cut to the chase.

I am a liar.

I have a darkness inside of me that I have hidden for, well, ever. It has taken me to the deepest, darkest corners of the human soul and left me wounded and broken in its wake. It never cared how I wanted to feel. In fact, it made me feel nothing at all, except in my daydreams. I spent years envisioning an icy-cool air embracing my body while I floated up into the clouds—where I could finally *feel* free.

How would I achieve this?

Well, the answer may be considered graphic, and I will activate the considerate trigger warning before proceeding.

Trigger warning.

I would fantasize about taking a knife to my wrists, slowly feeling the cool blade cut through my skin, allowing the blood to flow freely from my wrists and, with it, the pain.

Does that make me fucked up?

Quite possibly.

Now you can see why I have hesitated to tell this story for all these years. I have been terrified of how it would hurt not just me, but anyone involved. Anyone who might not have seen the pain, only that stupid fake smile I plastered all over my face while I was out in the world. Behind closed doors, I would spend my time lying in a ball on my floor, sobbing in the pitch black, and begging any god out there to take me away from this life.

Yes, I have given the gist, blabbed the highlights. Enough to be relatable, but not so much that the pain within my gut could be uncovered and brought to the surface.

I buried it for a reason.

Funny thing is that these things have a way of rising from the dead no matter how deep a grave you have dug to bury them.

To be honest, it is not funny at all.

It hurts.

My depression caused a pain so deep it bled into my body and provoked physical agony. For years, I could not even pinpoint the root cause of where this started. I knew the Thing was slowly killing me because I could not even admit that it occurred without being triggered and retraumatized. I spent years bargaining with a god to take the memories away, and when he would not do that, I decided to bury them myself.

But the impact that trauma has on you, especially when it goes untreated, is astronomical. It does not play fair, and it will not stay hidden. It creeps out into every aspect of your life. It expresses itself in the form of intense mistrust towards yourself and everyone around you.

It expresses itself in seemingly laughable fears that overwhelm your capacity to rationalize your way through them. It leaves you broken, bleeding, paralyzed, confused, and any other uncomfortable adjective that you can think of; it leaves you there.

People would tell me,

"Don't let this ruin your life."

But they were too late. It already had.

Somehow, I found my way to therapy and summoned an invisible courage to raise the dead. Therapy makes you peel the onion and find its core. If you think an onion burns and your eyes water uncontrollably as you cut through the layers, try unveiling psychological trauma and learning how to live with that.

I had been peeling layers back for nearly a year before I decided that I could muster the strength to write down my experiences. I hope my story can give words to those who may not have the courage or even desire to speak their own. I hope to share with you, who may be struggling, or you, who has a loved one on the brink of a nervous breakdown, why suicide seems like the best option—and, most importantly, why it is not.

I will say that one more time: it is not.

If I say I am sharing my journey from darkness to *light*, that would be another lie, so I will say *mostly light*, in hopes that it will encourage you to either ask for help or offer your help. To draw attention to topics so taboo that most of us fake our happiness. To bring assurance that living does not have to be unbearable, and that you can find purpose in your pain.

That there can be joy after trauma. And that your story, no matter how ordinary, can prove to be powerful.

That you can survive and subsequently thrive.

I did.

Maybe it does not matter.

But I am here anyway.

IDLE OF DESPAIR

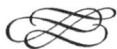

H i, my name is Sara.

I have been diagnosed with obsessive compulsive disorder, generalized anxiety disorder, post-traumatic stress disorder, depression and postpartum depression.

If *"you are messed up"* were a diagnosis, it would be easier to say and use fewer characters.

Oh, sorry, I use my twisted sense of humor when discussing topics that make my skin crawl. So, let us talk. Let us face the mental illness stigma by giving it a big ol' middle finger, shall we?

I have sought treatment for the last twenty-one years in the form of therapy and, more recently, prescription medications. They are used to balance the chemicals in my brain as well as lessen the physical manifestations of anxiety that I experience on a daily basis. These include palpitations, chest pain, shortness of breath, regular and vivid nightmares, the inability to quiet my mind once a fearful thought enters it, and the subsequent behaviors I adopt in an attempt to bring that oh-so-desperately-sought-after silence.

I fall prey to a panic attack several times a month. What does that feel like? Like I described a few pages ago, but here is a refresher: legit like I am dying. All the above symptoms with uncontrollable tears and all-consuming abdominal pain and nausea and even vomiting at times, which is its own form of cruelty because there is nothing I hate more than a queasy stomach.

Frequently, I hear, "I don't know how you do it."

And I cringe.

There is a misconception that I have it all together.

False.

I do things to keep my mind busy. Long ago, I realized that my quiet mind led to my loud, obnoxious, anxious thoughts. I think of myself as having good days and bad days. On the bad days I can barely find the inner strength to start my morning. The thought of my body moving forward seems impossible. My mind tends to go down a deep, dark rabbit hole that leads me to paralyzing fear and complete devastation. I have been known to succumb to irrational fears and overwhelming sadness that disguises itself as nothingness.

There is no greater blessing than the health of my children, and I know it. I know my worth. I know I am lucky to wake up and be given the opportunity to face another day. I know that there are people struggling with "real" problems. However, I am tired of pretending that mental illness is not one of them.

I get up. Through the grace of God. Through determination. Through the tiny voices that wake me up with, "Can I 'nuggle you, Momma?"

I keep going. Even when it feels impossible.

As does everyone who chooses to keep fighting whatever demons they are facing.

Although I sound confident and ready to tackle a system

that is filled with prejudice—one that attaches stigma to mental illness—I must admit that I have hesitated to do it. There are people who will use this frankness against me. They will question my sanity. They will invalidate my emotions. They will question my abilities. They will call me names. In short, I am a scaredy-cat.

I am doing what I am supposed to be doing; I go to counseling and take my medications; I do yoga and journal and make time for Jesus. Yet sometimes depression finds me, and sometimes that is because I am a busy middle-class working mom of five who occasionally runs out of time, often runs out of money, and tends to run out of memory.

About two and a half weeks ago, I last saw my psychiatrist. I happen to like this physician. He seems to make it a point to use the allotted fifteen minutes to its fullest. He follows up on all previous complaints. Of course, he is looking down at his notes from the last session to do so, but I appreciate the effort. There is just one tiny flaw to his care: written prescriptions. He will only refill prescriptions at office visits. I get it: discourage drug-seeking behavior and perhaps encourage responsibility among patients. But what the system does not seem to account for is head-full, memory-short, sleep-deprived mothers who take the prescription, remember putting it in their wallet and saying to themselves, "You put it in your wallet," only to find out there is no such prescription in said wallet.

And then you remember that maybe you actually put it in your back jeans pocket.

You run to the closet and start sliding your hand into all the pockets of all the pants you own. Empty. And then you remember that you saw it on your kitchen counter, and you said out loud, "Oh there it is, better not lose it," and yet here you are with a lost prescription and out of medications.

The consequences of such a loss include feeling strangely tight in my chest—almost like my heart is pounding in there, yet my heart rate is slow and regular. My head aches and my stomach turns. I am tired. No, exhausted. I usually supplement with alprazolam to try and calm my nerves. Every sound near me sounds like an explosion going off. I am slightly off balance, maybe dizzy, but more like my brain is outside my body and I am just floating. I cannot quite focus on any task at hand. I cannot fall asleep, nor can I keep my eyes open. But, boy, do they burn. Human touch provokes an unbearable need to scream. I cannot take it. I need space. I feel a ball of anger in the pit of my stomach that is making its way up my esophagus to the top of my throat. I become completely overwhelmed and frustrated. I leave messages with my doctor and ask if someone can phone in a refill, or at the very least if I can come by and pick up another prescription. I have called my pharmacy and asked them to contact my doctor's office for my much-needed refill. It is not a controlled medication, surely they have those rules for opioids and benzos—not your run-of-the mill antidepressants? But what if they will not provide a prescription? I am not supposed to just stop these medications, I am supposed to wean off them.

The awful symptoms of missing two days of medications take their toll. I become irritable, anxious and physically ill. My body feels like it is itching from the inside out. I want to peel my skin back and scratch or rub or soothe these tingling-in-the-worst-ways areas. I find myself being angry that my mind requires medication to alter its chemicals to function in my world. Why won't my body produce its own serotonin and make it readily available? The thought of stopping my medications is tempting to me. Do I really need these mood-altering drugs? Being dependent on pills to keep my brain operating at an average capacity?

It never fails that I run out of medication or I forget a day, and then I feel it. And it almost feels worse than the endless hole of darkness. Or maybe it does not. It all feels bad; I do not think I can compare. Surely, I can battle this disease sans medication. Surely, I do not need capsules to stay alive. Surely, I am strong enough to find my way to the light if I succumb to the darkness. Or do I only feel equipped to do so because I am on medication that balances my brain? Staying afloat with counseling alone: can I? Does Prozac make me worse? I cannot live like this—missing my dose a couple days and rendered helpless.

I feel the darkness. That is it I will just stop taking it and battle mental illness with diet, exercise and counseling. Oh, the counseling. That is breaking the bank, throwing a wrench in my budget. Maybe, I do not really need to go to counseling every month. Maybe, I can go every other month or just when I have a problem. I have some coping skills. I can implement them. Except when in the darkness; my compass then acts like I am in the Bermuda Triangle—spinning in circles without direction, unsure which way is home.

And I have been here before. Ready for battle. Putting my mental health aside to save money. To keep from feeling the lousy side effects of wearing off an SSRI. That leads me straight to unbearable pain. I feel trapped. I cannot live without these. I do not have enough financial stability to continue regular treatment. But what is life without emotional and mental stability? Without physical health? There is a saying that if you do not have your health, you do not have anything. That has to include mental health, right? I am worth my wellness, but sometimes I am frustrated that my wellness is so needy.

I find myself rushing through my hours, making sure everyone else has what they need to have a successful day, and in all my rushing I forget about what I need, for one. If I am being honest, my 90-day supply lasts somewhere near 180 to 270 days, which baffles my psychiatrist when I also assure him that I take my medications daily. I have never been good at math, so let us just say he can easily call my bluff with a calculator.

In terms of the counseling: at times I cancel appointments because something else comes up, like a sick child or a kid's wellness visit or lack of a babysitter, or my most favorite excuse: I am too depressed to go.

While I may be learning to recognize the signs that my mental illness is beginning to spiral out of control, first it had to spiral out of control. I suppose I had to hit a rock bottom of sorts and decide if I wanted to stay there, buried, or find my way back to the light. It is not easy to live like a human in an inhumane world, but through medication and counseling and meditation and yoga and distraction and a whole lot of determination, I am learning how to do just that.

And you know what I think?

I think you can too.

BROKEN SPIRIT

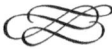

We moved back to the States when I was thirteen. It was a hard transition. I never quite felt American enough. Think *My Big Fat Greek Wedding.* I did not look American. I did not dress like American girls and boyfriends never happened for oh-so-many reasons—but the reason I am referring to now is parental rules due to cultural differences, or maybe just my dad's rules because he was a dad. I did not go to church; I was not quite Christian, but I was not Muslim either. I also was not really Arab, as I was not even fluent in the language. I never knew where my place was. To say I was an awkward teen is an understatement: crazy teeth, crazy hair. My sense of displacement led me to feel shy and insecure.

This seems as good a time as any to share a little of my testimony here. I know the idea of a supernatural being sent to save our souls can be cringe and eyeroll-worthy. I know that because I used to roll my eyes at the notion. But then I thought, so what? If that makes people feel whole and human and alive and hopeful, then how can it hurt? I guess it hurts when we stop using our faith as a moral compass and begin to use it as a way to justify hate.

I did my best to fit in where I could, but the past Thing would not leave me alone. I unraveled, fell apart, and never found my way back. I did not speak of the events for six years, but it consumed my every thought and invaded my every potential moment of happiness.

My days were spent going to school while my nights consisted of locking myself in my room and blaring the stereo to drown out the sound of my tears.

I would cry out to a higher power. Beg him to take these memories from me, bargaining with him to restore my innocence while questioning if I would make it to the Kingdom of Heaven or burn in the fires of Hell for what I'd let happen.

I had friends, but it was always on the forefront of my mind that if they knew my secret, then they would be disgusted by this shell of a human and cut off all ties. I was terrified of being left alone; I would avoid it whenever I could in an effort to keep my demons away.

Keeping secrets and writing them down became a habit. Going back through these words, I find that I betrayed myself even then.

This is where faith gets confusing.

My mom was sure Jesus was the Messiah and that I should accept him into my heart, and all my problems would dissipate. But only through churches with denominations with which she identified. Perhaps you know, but Christianity has way too many paths to Jesus. You can pretty much find a church that has tailored its views to match your own.

Nevertheless, my dad was always there to counter that fact and instill doubt because our Savior was yet to come. I would try to go to church, but my dad was not keen on that idea. To be fair, he also did not want me to go to Mosque. You see, my dad is against established religion. He is philosophical and theoretical, and for a broken mind of teenage proportions that does not settle well.

I feel that this would be as good a time as any to talk about Islam. After all, it will become more relevant as the story continues.

While living overseas in Kuwait, because my father was Muslim, I was required to take religion class. That religion was obviously Islam. I spent five years learning the faith and the daily prayers. I was never once encouraged to hurt or harm anyone. I was taught a religion of peace, one for which Jesus was a prophet, but not the son of God, so the Messiah still had to make his debut to our suffering souls. One in which we worshiped the same God as our Christian counterparts, just in a different way. As a result, we were taught that we must earn our way into heaven. Through our actions. These actions include sacrificing literal lambs, fasting during Ramadan, praying at certain times of the day. Since the Lamb of God was yet to be, we were responsible for requesting forgiveness to our own sins.

And we are back to my teenage, self-loathing self. Case in point is the journal entry below.

Tuesday, February 15, 2000
Second month of 2000, and it has gone by fast. I have not even stuck to my resolution. I have so many feelings to write about, so here I go. I want to be thin. Flat stomach and all. I have lost weight, but I still binge. I need to look DEEP inside me and find self-control. It is unbelievably hard though—you have no idea! Yesterday I came home and just ate, and I hated me so

much. And I HATE hating me because I have to be there for me when no one else is, and I failed myself yesterday. I just wanted to cry every time I walked past a mirror.

Oh, did I mention I struggled with food, and my relationship to it was on the rocks for quite some time?

In fact, I have spent most of my life battling food in one manner or another. I suppose now is the time to sum up those struggles for you and really paint the picture of what my disordered eating habits have looked like.

As a teen, the battle consisted of avoiding food for the purpose of punishing myself. They say withholding food is an eating disorder, one that is about control. If that is true, then I was trying to control my perception of myself. I was filled with self-hatred because... trauma.

I drew the conclusion that I was not worthy of, well, anything. And since my insides were broken and bleeding amidst the turmoil, I placed value on my outsides.

Flat stomachs, thin waistlines, sunken cheekbones, visible collar bones: all were conduits of happiness.

My meals would consist of four *Triscuits* and half a cup of orange juice—until I could not take it anymore. The overwhelming nausea resulting from intense hunger pangs would take control. Like a raccoon scavenging through the trash, I would cave and indulge in any and all foods I could find. Until my stomach felt swollen and my spirit defeated.

I was as worthless as I'd always known I was.

Truthfully, I do not know what flipped the switch in my mind. One day I thought that four crackers and juice did not make a meal. I decided to cure myself, and I began to eat whatever I wanted, whenever I wanted.

But my body had other plans.

My anxieties became more intense, and my stomach became weaker. It came to a point when I could not tolerate any foods other than prepackaged *Rice Krispy* treats, saltine crackers, and water. The more kids I had, the more I would be complimented: *"You don't look like you've had kids."*

And all I could think was, *"You would look like this too if you couldn't eat."*

But I would smile and say, *"Thanks, I don't get much time to sit and eat these days."*

Although I was hurting, I would feel a slight sense of pride for being able to function without food and that the shape of my body reflected it.

They would smile and nod in what appeared to be a silent understanding among strangers and reply, *"You have your hands full."*

True, but my mind was fuller.

After multiple emergency room visits for excruciating abdominal pain—in danger to be labeled a drug seeker—ruined and canceled vacations with family, and an inpatient stay, I underwent all the testing determined appropriate by a gastroenterologist.

I was eventually diagnosed with Irritable Bowel Syndrome (IBS). This is also known as a diagnosis of exclusion, meaning there is no other explanation for my symptoms. You see, as a healthcare provider, I knew what IBS meant.

I was crazy.

Insert your friendly sarcastic tone here.

I remember the physician assistant telling me, *"We don't know why, but for some reason those with IBS have a sensitive GI tract. They can feel everything moving through their intestines."*

No idea whether she was trying to make me feel like my

diagnosis was legitimate or whether it is true, but I nodded and once again felt conquered.

They tried a medication to interrupt the signal between my stomach and brain, but all it did was make me sleep away my days, and with young children to care for I needed to be awake.

I began to realize that there probably was nothing actually wrong with me, except my head. But when food makes you sick—in a real or imagined condition—it becomes hard to eat.

I developed a fear of food. Since I never knew what food would lead to pain that would knock me to my knees, I never wanted to eat. I would consume enough to dull the hunger pangs and subdue the nausea. I was always wary of pain, and somehow this transitioned into a fear of making food that would poison my family.

Meal preparation became very difficult, as did eating out. I did not trust food. I marked certain foods as safe with no rhyme or reason, other than the fact that I could tolerate them. We ate lots of fruits and vegetables, until all of those became contaminated with E. coli and at some point recalled.

SIDE NOTE: Recalls render me incapacitated and desperately searching for another safe food to take its place.

Cooking raw meat from scratch was impossible. If something did not *feel* like it had frozen correctly or defrosted properly, it would end up in the trash. I am not sure what right *feels* like; nevertheless, the monetary value of food that I threw in the trash due to overwhelming fear was, I am sure, astronomical.

Sorry, environment.

My husband was always there to reassure me that feeding my family was the right thing to do. That nutritious food was not the enemy. Yes, the man is an actual saint. I started having him smell all the foods before I cooked them, examine them with me to ensure he did not see some invisible plague that would ravage our intestines and take our children from us.

It took years to admit this fear in counseling. I did not know how to say it.

I just say prayers before preparing foods and beg God to keep my family healthy.

And safe.

I ask him to help me distinguish between reality and my mind being an evil liar. To help me believe what my husband is telling me: that I am not poisoning my family.

Things have been better since I found a working antidepressant and an anti-anxiety medication that calms my brain and subsequently my actions. It makes cooking food easier. To form new opinions and expand the options of what I deem safe. To tell my mind that food is nourishment and not poison.

Nourishment that I need to function.

As I started eating more, I started feeling better.

I also started gaining weight.

A lot of it.

I stopped weighing myself when the scales tipped over thirty pounds of weight gain.

For someone who has placed value on thinness, it was hard to accept.

I had to decide that numbers are liars and not an accurate representation of my health.

Or worth.

If they were, then my non-eating, internally decomposing self was a "healthy" weight, and all the therapy I have had since to redefine my worth has been wrong.

TO CLARIFY: That is also sarcasm.

Yes, the pounds piled on. My clothing sizes went up, my face became fuller.

Despite exercise and listening to hunger cues, my size increased. Truthfully, that part has been a process of learning to accept my body in its "as is" condition.

I am thankful for counseling to remind me that I am worthy of being me, and that my hunger is not a weakness. That I do not need to punish myself for emotionally crippling wounds I experienced as a child. That my worth is not reduced by stretch marks and cellulite.

I am not going to lie—there are still foods I refuse to eat. They led to such excruciating pain that I have no desire to experiment. I do not know if they are an actual intolerance or were the result of a mind seeped in invisible pain.

But the victory is that now I eat. And I feed my family with less guilt and fear than I had before. And the realization that my larger size does not mean a smaller worth.

Yes, I give myself pep talks daily and implement the coping skills I have learned in therapy.

They work.

I am healing.

But it is work.

My battles with trauma, subsequent damaged self-image, and lack of self-esteem took their toll on my fragile mind. This usually takes the form of hopelessness and looking for a way out. There never seems to be one, so I look for a way that may not make sense to others but seems completely viable to me: suicide.

I considered suicide twice as a teen. The first time occurred after I went to my room for a typical all-out crying sesh. I was home alone, and I walked up our stairs as I had so many times before. But this time was different. When I reached the top of the stairs to make that immediate right turn into my bedroom, I was met with resistance. Both figurative and literal, if you will.

My door may have been open, but there was a wall blocking me from entering. It felt as if the tears and pain I had released into this space had never left and were now taking up all the space. I could not enter. And I wept. Because now I really had nowhere to go, and now I just had to be done.

Returning to the kitchen area of our home, I grabbed a steak knife. I felt my heart pounding with relief. I laid the steel against the skin on my wrist as I had fantasized so many times before. I placed the knife on my wrists, and in an instant I had a flash forward to my two younger brothers, who were ten and five at the time, walking in to find my blood-soaked corpse lying on the floor. Although I longed for the release, I heard a quiet voice tell me that they would not recover from a trauma like this, and that I should not give up and keep going in this life with the promise that it would get better.

I dropped the knife and fell to my knees. Because now I really was trapped. Trapped in a life I did not know how to live, consumed by terror that would not leave, filled with sorrow that had no release and with the painful feeling that I had nowhere to go.

Ideation number two came after I had gone to a Sunday morning mass. I have always been drawn to Catholicism and was never quite sure why. Perhaps it is the dominant denomination in the Gateway to the West. Or maybe it was God calling me to provide me with the structure of faith that my life was so clearly lacking. Either way, church was painful. It hurt because I did not know what to believe. I did not know if I was going to hell if I could not accept Jesus, or if I was going anyway because I was a dirty human being with a disgusting past. I just did not know.

One day, the unknown became unbearable. I came home to a father who was angry at me for attending church. I was more confused than ever. I went to my room with a bottle of Tylenol and a pad of paper. I honestly did not know if it would end my pain, but I was banking on the fact that it would. I began to write my goodbye letter, explaining to my family why I had to leave. My tears flowed because there was a little voice deep down inside that did not want me to go, but a louder one telling me I just could not stay. At that moment, my mom knocked on my door. She talked to me, hugged me, and whatever conversation we might have had, I do not remember. Except one thing. She said, "I'll talk to your dad so you can go to church." That brought some light into my darkness, and I decided I would keep going.

I never told her that, and I suspect that if she does choose to read this book this is the first she is hearing of it. I do not know if she had an intuition that said *knock,* but if she did and followed it: Mom, thank you.

Suicide was off the table for many years. A tiny voice would whisper to me that things would get better. I would find myself filling with rage and beg the voice to stop lying. I did not want the promise of false hope when I knew hope was a fairytale. Still, I chose life. Not one that brought me joy, but I chose to keep breathing until I could not. That is the thing about demons. If you do not battle them head on and completely, they will find their way back to you.

More on that later.

I have always wondered if my depression was a result of my brain chemicals being changed by the trauma I endured. Or if I was depressed anyway. I will never know if my mental illness has been shaped by circumstances outside of my control or by genetics, or a combination of everything.

I always want to believe that it is genetics. The hand I was dealt. Because accepting the idea that a trauma provoked by someone else's decision changed the course of my life in ways I would not have chosen, altered the wirings of my brain—to give them that kind of power...

... I cannot.

So, I tell myself I would have had depression no matter what. It just stole my joy before I knew how to find it.

BATTLING DEMONS

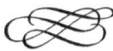

Tuesday, September 29, 1998, 4:05 p.m.

Yesterday *I tore out about 7-10 entries, and I feel so much better now! They were just so depressing, and I am not depressed! I feel like a huge weight has been lifted from my chest.*

Thursday, September 2, 1999

I am feeling a bit depressed today, so please bear with me. Actually, I have been feeling this way since school started. I feel so unloved, unwanted, and alone. Those, in my opinion, are the worst things to feel, especially all at once. And what I hate even more is they are becoming stronger every day, and there is absolutely nothing I can do to stop it. I have tried really hard, but it is not working. And I know life is what you make it, but I KNOW I am not doing this to me. I wouldn't want to put myself through this much pain and depression.

. . .

Actual journal entries. I have always written to process my pain and discomfort. In my teens, the literal loneliness that ensued caused true physical pain. I could feel it in my heart. The way it would ache. The salt in my tears made my eyes tingle while they overwhelmed my ducts until they silently fell down my cheeks. My throat would burn from holding back the quiet sobs. I would wake up each morning and look into the mirror at my red, swollen face. It threatened to betray me and announce to the world that my tears had fallen all night. I would do what I could to calm my telltale face with warm showers and cold sink water.

And now, I have a journal in my nightstand drawer that makes me cringe. It is a necessary evil. I only bring it out when I am on the verge of a mental breakdown. Like when I want to utilize all the unhealthy coping mechanisms. The writing is ferocious and sloppy and vulnerable, which leads to embarrassment when my mind has taken its chill pill and calmed down a smidge. I keep it buried under a pile of books, drawer closed, and it feels like it threatens me with its mere presence. It is another dirty little secret I have, and my insides would melt and dissolve if my kids or husband read it. Come to think of it, it should have a lock and chains to ensure the contents remain hidden until my very last breath. And then get buried with me.

What could be so embarrassing, you ask.

It reminds me that I am broken. An actual broken human struggling to maintain composure on a daily basis. Sometimes it feels like that is who I really am. I tend to describe myself as broken and bleeding, and my journal really reinforces that narrative. It gets me thinking though. I am broken. We all are. Isn't that kind of lovely? We keep wanting to pretend we are okay, and I just do not know if we are.

Then it gets me thinking even more: isn't that the whole

point of Jesus? Isn't that why we need him? My journey to finding a solid faith has been anything but easy, but it makes me feel better to know that I am not the only broken human in a fractured world.

The closest my tears ever came to calling me out was during my teen years. My dad said to me, "When I look at you, it makes me sad because all I see is the pain in your eyes."

That was the most seen I ever was.

Until May 2019.

"*Mom, why are you making that face?*" So asks my five-year-old while we are driving home from the grocery store.

"*What face?*" I ask, unaware.

"*This one.*" She scowls, demonstrating.

"*Oh, I'm just thinking,*" I reply.

"*I make that face when I'm thinking too. When I'm thinking sad thoughts.*"

My heart breaks. Because my daughter knows sad thoughts, and I wonder if that is how it starts. And because I, at that moment, am planning my suicide.

I call my husband. "*I have to tell you something when I get home, and if I don't say it now, then I don't know what will happen. Tell the kids to go play.*"

That is a lie. I know what will happen; he will be planning a funeral.

At that moment, I could not see any positive purpose in my existence. Only pain and suffering for myself and those around me because of my depression. I will be lightening their load, truly. I am constantly surrounded by my children and husband, and yet I feel so completely alone. They have no idea who I am on the inside. To be honest, neither do I. I am not sad, yet I cannot stop the tears. I am not angry, but I am always yelling. I am not sleepy, but I just want to stay in bed all day.

I am empty.

Confused.

Alone.

Lonely.

Dark.

My mind and body do not merge. They seem to be completely separate entities existing in parallel dimensions to one another. I am not whole, just broken. It hurts. Unbearable pain that has nowhere to go. Confined by the structure that is my skeleton. It is building inside me, and I cannot get it out. I want so badly to open my body and breathe; let the pain escape. To feel it leaking slowly into the seemingly endless open space around me.

I begin to choke on my words. If I say it out loud, I have to deal with the consequences. I want to say: I am going to kill myself. Saturday night while you are out. Bathtub so as not to make a mess. After the kids are asleep. I will lock the door so that only you can open it to find me. Picturing the blood flowing from my wrist wounds is a relief. All pain leaking out. I cannot live anymore. I do not know why or how. Everything feels too much. I am drowning. I cannot breathe. I am being sucked into a black hole of darkness. I have lost my direction, my vision. Honestly, in this moment, I do not want to die; I just cannot live like this.

But I cannot say that. So, I cheat.

"I have been thinking of ways to kill myself."

I do not know why I told him, but I did. All the while, my voice cracked. I am shaking. Trembling. Terrified. I do not want to say the words. Are they even true? Is this who I am now? Is this real?

He looks at me with concern in his eyes, a poker face on.

Lying in bed, hands folded calmly on his chest. I can see he is listening.

He opens his arms. "Come here."

The tears begin to flow, I am sobbing. Cannot catch my breath. Everything is blurry.

I know he told me not to go anywhere. He said we would get help. I told him I did not want anyone to know. What will people think? They are going to say they told me not to have so many kids. That it is too much. They are going to say they knew I could not handle it. Whatever *it* is. They are going to say they told me so. They are going to say they had no idea and that I do not have any reasons to be sad. To just think positively and I will feel better. Exercise, it will go away. Take time for yourself, and you will be rejuvenated. Is this real?

Honestly, I do not know how I got here. I thought I was taking care of myself. I guess I was not. I had been doing everything I was supposed to do. Taking my medicine and doing yoga. Trying to get in for counseling appointments, but they always seem to take a back seat to sick kids or sick me. It is not working. I am always numb and forever hurting at the same moment.

I cannot make any decisions. I cannot answer any questions. We go to see my counselor, my psychiatrist. They want to know what my trigger was. What sent me to this moment of daydreaming of suicide and cutting. Everyone wants to know why. Everyone wants to blame it on something. Work, extracurricular activities, kids, life. I cannot pinpoint a trigger. This has been boiling inside of me for months.

No, years.

I have actively been telling myself "I'll deal with it later." Never knowing when later would be, but apparently it is now. I knew I was heading to a point of no return when I saw

A Star Is Born, the new one with Bradley Cooper and Lady Gaga. We watched it, and SPOILER ALERT: Bradley Cooper's character commits suicide. When that scene flashed across my screen, I thought: "He's lucky it's over."

Recently I came across a black and white internet square image. On the left side of the image was a simple curvy black line resembling a face profile. Inside the silhouette were the words "help me" written over and over, top to bottom, left to right, filling the face. The right side of the square was white and blank, with two words written near the mouth of the face: "I'm fine." And that is who I was from 1992-2019. Fine.

It may or may not surprise some to hear that even when planning my suicide, I did not want the finality of death. I remember thinking I wish I could bleed out all this pain and then be back to my old self again. Death was just collateral damage.

For me, it was about needing out. Unable to bear the pain. I have never drowned, but I imagine depression being in a state of constant, eternal drowning. You cannot breathe, but so desperately crave air. Lungs burning, lips parted trying to bring in oxygen but met with an intense resistance. Giving anything to be able to feel the sweet relief of your head surfacing above the waters and yet never being able to rise. For me, suicide was about coming up for air.

Eighteen years had passed between the last time I seriously considered suicide. The thoughts would come to my mind, and I would respond that there were better ways to cope. Until one day I could not. I felt it coming on for about a year; that is what prompted me to seek psychiatric help. And I thought it helped, but I guess it was not enough. I was not going to counseling enough—I think I have made it clear how that happened: life. I lost sight of the light and became consumed by darkness. It came so fast; all of a sudden, here we were. Back in the counselor's office, the psychiatrist's office, being told that I needed more treatment. That we needed to keep me safe. That I was worth the life I was given.

It all seems so petty, but I assure you that the depth of the darkness is no joke. It does not leave any cracks for light to peek in. It is all consuming and literally painful. It hurts, and I just wanted it to feel better.

I went to intensive outpatient therapy three times a week, saw a psychiatrist once a week (and went through an array of medication changes). I also saw my individual counselor once every other week.

I am lucky.

Lucky because external forces—I call those forces God—gave me the strength to mutter, "help." Not everyone can say the same. And I wonder how many people are dying because of it.

HASHTAG-ME-TOO

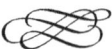

"I never feel safe," I tell my husband as I sob uncontrollably after a counseling session. I had to call him from work to leave early and come pick me up. "You told me to call you if I felt like I couldn't live. I can't."

"Hang on, I'm coming to get you."

The effects of the Thing have haunted me for the last twenty-seven years. Always finding new ways to remind me that it happened. You think you deal with it. You think you have healed and moved on. You think you have not let it define you. And then your son's new body spray is eerily familiar, and you are back there, unable to remove yourself from the situation. Wishing to God it was all a nightmare. Frantically finding all clothing with that disgusting scent and shoving it into the washer. Washing it over and over to ensure that you never have to smell it ever again. You take his cologne and throw it away while he is at school because you cannot bear to even look at it. And you definitely cannot bear to have your child be a trigger for your overwhelming pain.

And then you wonder what you are supposed to do with

that. You wonder how you are supposed to distinguish between the past and now when so many things take you right back. Not necessarily back to the actions that occurred, but back to the feelings. When you felt trapped, terrified, alone. When you would want to scream but you were paralyzed. When the fear and disgust were overwhelming. Where deep regret lives. You thank God that you have a counseling appointment and you hope you are strong enough to mention it then. But more than that, you hope you are strong enough to deal with the repercussions of speaking this truth. Because talking about it is also a trigger.

I first went to a counselor when I was eighteen. She was very...

... clinical.

So I dumped her. I then tried a multitude of therapists, none of whom I jived with. To all I would have to repeat my trauma and then leave their office more wounded and bloodied than when I'd entered. I could not yet overcome it. At the time I first sought counseling, I had told a handful of people what had happened to me. The fear of being labeled disgusting and rejected as a human was far too great for me to be able to speak of this freely. I buried it again until I was twenty-three and expecting my first child.

My husband and I were going through what you might call a rough phase. Mostly exacerbated by the fact that his wife, me, was ill equipped to handle her past and her emotions. She was truly a shattered human being. Still is, but I am slowly starting to glue myself back together. But that girl, she hated herself. And life. And him. She hated everyone for not understanding how afraid she was. How she always held her head low and wanted to be invisible. Never wanting to draw any attention to herself that could turn into another tragedy. She was not sure how to live, and she was quite certain that if she were not pregnant she would fix that problem. She would scream at her husband, throw things, trying desperately to clear an internal pain that refused to release her exhausted spirit. Until, finally, she could feel her baby move and realized that a person was coming, and this person deserved a better mother than her.

So, she asked her obstetrician for help, and he gave her the name of a counselor. Whom, fifteen years later, she still sees.

When I first met my counselor and once again unveiled my pain and she threw her "put it in a box" wisdom at me, I was deep in darkness, seeped in pain and entrenched in regret.

Still begging God to make me forget it ever happened.

Maybe your story does not include coping with personal trauma, but I am willing to bet it includes managing global ones. I don't know about you, but I feel like the world has been on fire since forever. While I have not found a way to squelch the flames, I am hell bent on smoldering the hate that fuels them.

SEMICOLONS AND CIRCLES

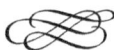

September 11, 2001.

Depending on your generation, that date elicits different things for different people. I remember the overwhelming fear of what that attack would mean for my family. For starters, it meant being inspected more thoroughly at airports than my fair-skinned counterparts; despising terrorism as much as they did had no bearing on how I was viewed. One time I was searched because I packed a toothbrush, and did you know that toothbrushes look like weapons on bag scanners?

I place my bags on the scanner at the airport. The security officer looks at the screen and then looks at me suspiciously. I stare back.

"There is something concerning in your bag."

Huh? I look at the screen: clothes, a hairdryer is clearly delineated, toiletries. She must have noticed I was confused.

"This, here." She points to a toothbrush.

"Um, that is my toothbrush."

"We have to be sure."

They take me to the side and pat me down; all clear. I am

allowed to take my bags and continue through security. Maybe she really believed it was a weapon. Or maybe my last name gave me away. My maiden name, Khuraibet (Kur-ray-bet), has led many people to ask me where I am really from.

Our honeymoon took place in Jamaica.

We landed and proceeded through security; the officer looked at my passport. It still had my maiden name on it.

"Where are you from?" he says in the local accent.

"The States."

"No, where are you from?" he repeats.

I knew what he was getting at, but I did not feel like explaining, yet again, my background.

"St. Louis."

"No, this." He points to my last name. "Where are you from?" He emphasizes his words.

"My last name is from Kuwait."

"What are you doing here?"

"On my honeymoon." I motion towards my new husband.

He looks me over, hands my passport back and lets me through.

I must say, traveling with my married Eastern European name definitely makes things simpler.

I remember my father becoming an American. He fought in the War on Terror for four years. He gave more than most American-born individuals, myself included. He returned only to be questioned. He has said on many occasions that he will play into the terrorist jokes. He should not have to.

In my mind, his absence was the beginning of the end for my parents. As an adult, you begin to realize that your idealistic childhood view may have been skewed. They were separated for far too long. He fought for his country, and it feels like his reward was the demise of our family. He returned to a country consumed by prejudice. He always said America was the greatest country, and yet it treated him as though he was an enemy. In case you are wondering, he no longer lives in the United States; he moved back to Kuwait to start a new life. One in which I know he will not encounter the hate he did in "the land of the free."

Individuals have long "joked" with my husband that he is "sleeping with the enemy." These remarks have always been bothersome. After all, I am American. I condemn terrorism. I want to stop hate and promote tolerance. But I am supposed to laugh and "not take it personally."

You know what, it is personal—and it is just not funny.

Fast-forward several years to the present day. I am left wondering where the line will be drawn. How far will people go to squelch their fear? I may be American, but I have Arab blood and Muslim ties—aka, family and friends—as do my children. I know our country has a history of reacting to fear with confinement. After all, Japanese Americans were placed in internment camps during World War II. Every time I hear, "history repeats itself," I pray with every ounce of my being that it is not repeated in the confinement of Arab-Americans.

I can hide behind the ignorance: people think I am either Italian, Mexican or Hispanic. I do not have an accent, so when I am asked: "Where are you from?"

And I answer: "Here."

They accept it. Not every immigrant or person of color has that luxury.

Today I am free, but it is in the back of my mind that it may not always be. If I am being honest, I am discouraged by the number of people who still view Muslims as terrorists instead of understanding that terrorists are criminals.

When I share my life experiences, the usual response is, "That's not how it is."

"You are an American; no one is hateful towards you."

"No one behaves that way. That doesn't happen."

If only that were true. However, it is not. People unknowingly—at times innocently, other times purposefully—dismiss the reality of my world and the world of countless others.

My Arab roots, giving people the green light to pass judgment and direct hate towards me.

I am here to say that it happens.

I am also here to say that it does not have to.

I would like to believe that my experiences have helped shape an empathetic heart with the potential to bring awareness to the hatefulness and struggles that exist in our world and so in the winter of 2018, I became a mental health advocate. I had been dabbling in philanthropy for about a year and a half when I found another human with a desire to help others the way I longed to do. Together we formed a grassroot nonprofit that we named *Love Will Foundation*. We settled on this name because we are determined to show what love will do when we try. Along the way, a dandelion became an unofficial part of our logo and our mission because where some see weeds, we see wishes.

Our nonprofit is operated by selfless volunteers who find passion in our mission. We fundraise practically every month of the year so that we can pay for as many counseling sessions as possible that we then donate. We recently did some math and discovered that to date (2023), we are approaching $25,000 of financial assistance for counseling sessions in the Saint Louis area—which is where we are based. I wish that number were two million, but, alas, even one dollar matters.

I did not really think through the whole "mental health

advocate" thing when I decided to become one, but apparently talking about mental health comes with the territory. And when you talk about mental health and have mental illness, the two are bound to intertwine. I started getting asked "why mental health," and I slowly started to leak out the fact that it was because I know how hard it is to find counseling and how much harder to afford it.

And how it should not be that way.

Along this journey, I discovered the semicolon and what it means within the mental health community. For those that do not know, the semicolon indicates when an author could have ended a sentence but instead decided to continue it. If you have struggled with any form of mental illness, then you probably know that sometimes it can be quite challenging to keep your story going. To not say *The End* with a definite, forceful, and irreversible period.

I am an author, a trauma survivor, and a mental illness warrior. As such, I have become familiar with punctuation. When it comes to writing, I have a hard time not forming run-on sentences filled with semicolons. When it comes to battling depression, flashbacks, anxiety, and triggers, sometimes I have a hard time not using that infamous period.

But I made a promise to my husband the day that I confessed my inner demons. A promise that I would keep going. A promise I was not sure I would be able to keep. I have often wondered if I will succumb to my illness. Will I fight all these battles only to lose the war?

For a long time, I was unsure. So, I had to find a way to remind myself of the promise I made. And so I had that silly semicolon tattooed on my body, and from the semicolon circle birds are flying to their freedom.

Because I want to be free. Free from the intrusive thoughts that swirl in my brain. Free from the incessant noise that comes with constant panic. Free from the nothing that depression forces upon me.

Once I completed my intensive outpatient therapy program and actually believed the promise I had made, I had my tattoo completed. Into a circle. With a dandelion. Where the seeds merge with the birds. Because a dandelion, you see, is all about perspective. To some, it is a weed—but I have always blown those white fluffy seeds into the wind, and as each one sails away, so does a wish that I have attached to it. That is not a metaphorical coincidence, my friends. No. It is my reminder. A reminder that mental illness may want to end my story, but when depression sees a period, I choose to see a semicolon.

Ah, sweet perspective.

STILL STANDING

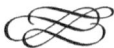

"*I can see the light in you. Sara is back,*" my therapist said at a counseling session following the completion of my intensive outpatient therapy program. And I felt it too. God, it felt good.

Although it is a little strange to make peace with death, yearn for relief, and then find yourself still alive. And wanting to live. But I have been grateful for the chance.

I was determined to think I was strong enough to handle this disease without anyone's help. I fooled myself into thinking that my medications were optional. I completed thirteen sessions of intensive outpatient therapy when I realized that mental illness is real and requires outside intervention.

I have now accepted and learned that asking for help is not a weakness. Neither is the row of prescriptions that line my cabinet. It is not a secret of which to be ashamed. It is part of managing this chronic illness, which is a chemical imbalance.

The five weeks of my mental breakdown became a journey of healing and awareness. I learned *everything* from it. I do not feel the need to relive the past, but rather I am ready to move forward.

I have continued to practice my coping skills: being more mindful of my thoughts that turn into actions; taking my medications as prescribed; processing stressors as they happen; attending doctor and counseling appointments as indicated; and more.

Nine days after, my hope returned.

I felt better;

Lighter;

More capable;

Better prepared;

Ready;

I never thought I would, but I did. And I do.

To those who kept telling me my life was worth living...

... you were right;

SULTRY CIGARETTES

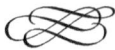

It wasn't too long ago that I walked into UPS to do the Amazon return thing, and on my way out I found a woman in late middle-age who was smoking.

Smoking.

In 2023.

And did I inhale the smoke eluding from her carbon monoxide byproduct because it smelled glorious and inviting? Yes. Yes, I did.

You see, I used to smoke. Sometimes I still do. It has been my unhealthy coping mechanism—easy button if you will—for a few years now. I started smoking when I was seventeen and found an old, open pack of cigarettes buried way up high in my parents' closet. And then I had a friend who was eighteen and I somehow had the balls to ask her to buy them for me until I was old enough to do the deed on my own.

I smoked through nursing school; that is right, as I was learning about the effects of nicotine and smoke inhalation on the brain and body, I sucked down cigarette after cigarette. Even more on study nights. My fellow nursing student friends and I would gather on the rooftop of our dorm, light up and discuss all the pulmonary diseases that smoking provoked.

Then I decided I wanted a baby and quit smoking while trying to get pregnant. It never really felt like a thing I had to quit or give up. I found myself sneaking into gas stations every now and again when I was not pregnant, and the stress was as great as the satisfaction of feeling smoke fill my lungs to the brim and the nicotine flow through my veins. It always made me nauseated and dizzy—it never made me feel better except for the moment I first lit up and soaked in that deep breath.

I returned to smoking circa late 2020. Yup. Pretty recently. I think we all know what it is about 2020 that provoked stress, so I will just give a quick trigger warning and mention that it was COVID.

And politics.

And vaccine debates.

And being in health care.

And watching people who were once running marathons not even being able to walk to their exam rooms sans oxygen and major panting because they had long-haul COVID.

And there being absolutely nothing that helped them.

I think an empath can only be empathetic for so long, and when we realize empathy is trivial and useless, we either fight harder or turn stone cold. I didn't have any fight left, so I became stone. I do not use the word hate lightly, but I hated everything about my profession and about people.

I burned out. I mean, crashed and burned. My capacity to cope was overwhelmed, so I turned to smoking. At first, I justified it. I needed it. It was the lesser of evils, meaning it was a way for me to self-harm without anyone actually knowing I was self-harming. I relished in it. Until my OB/GYN brought to my attention at a routine appointment that smoking at my age, especially if I needed any hormone replacement therapy (which I might), made me a high-risk person for blood clots.

First of all, rude.

Second, if coupled with the weight gains from getting older and reconditioning from COVID quarantines, he was right. I do not want to turn into the pulmonary patient that I have been caring for all these years. I bargained a bit with God to promise me that I could keep smoking without consequences.

He repetitively shot that down, and once I accepted that it was up to me to make good choices to have good outcomes, I smoked my last pack and put it down. So when I see someone smoking, I get jealous. I am jealous they had no need of that conversation or bargaining with their spiritual guide. I am envious that their desire to smoke outweighs their feels. I feel jealous that the threat of consequences weighs less for them than the distress of giving up smoking.

I like smoking. It gives me a release and a thrill that I often miss from my healthier coping mechanisms. It feels really good in the moment, and it makes me wish I could ride a lot of moments for longer without having to face reality. But I guess the thing I am learning is you really cannot escape reality. You cannot outrun life. You cannot stay in a singular moment forever. As trauma survivors, we have to recognize the moments pass; both the good ones and the bad ones.

It won't always feel like this. It won't always make you want to quit. It won't always be too much to bear. That moment passes, and when it does you will be glad that you put down the thing that doesn't really help and opted for the thing that can spark some joy.

And that thing is hope.

LOVE, PTSD

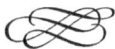

I'm sitting at my #4's Monday night sports practice; actually, I'm tucked away in the car to avoid being slammed in the head by rogue soccer balls because I'm not really in the mood for a concussion.

As I have a couple hours, I figure what better time to alleviate my brain of all the words saturating it. I have been thinking a lot lately about the whole idea of triggers and trigger warnings. After all, we live in an online world and have so much information at our fingertips. Not just information, but stories. And there is so much power in telling and listening to each other's stories. Truthfully, there's also pain. Especially when a story brings up emotions or memories that we are either not prepared to deal with or we have purposefully suppressed.

This is the kind of story that strips away my layers and makes me feel raw and vulnerable. I think the point of this whole book is that I am working on embracing these feelings, and so even when all the alarms sound off in my head to keep quiet, I have to fight through the urge and choose to speak up.

A few people may ask, "Why must you discuss such personal things? You should keep them private."

And that. That right there. That element of shame. That is why I do not. Because if I had spoken up sooner, then maybe this would not be my story, and maybe my words would let you know that you alone cannot carry the burden of your traumas.

Nor should you.

Enter 'trigger warnings.'

I see these on a lot of sites—especially blogs—where individuals are sharing past experiences.

Past *traumatic* experiences.

In fact, I see it so often that I feel like one could begin to just roll one's eyes at this overused terminology, and gloss over these oh-so-important words.

Trigger Warning. Let me tell you, as a person who struggles with PTSD, I hold on to these warnings like I hold on to the Gospel.

The part that is hard about participating in an online world (*and maybe that is one of the major reasons social media provoked my anxiety, now that I am thinking about it*) is reading or watching or reliving someone's trauma. It is, well, traumatizing. Especially when *you* are recovering from one or more traumatic events.

It is also hard to live in a real-life world where you can be minding your own business, living your own life, and a trigger unexpectedly and rudely takes hold of you. Something as simple as a book—that has nothing to do with you or your trauma, mind you—can be a trigger.

In fact, that happened to me yesterday. I was reading the loveliest book, and all of a sudden I was gone.

What does that mean? I do not know if all people with PTSD who find themselves suddenly taken back to unpleasant memories feel this way, but I will attempt to describe what it physically and mentally is like to be triggered.

My eyes sting and burn with the threat of tears, but I cannot actually cry. My stomach is in knots, and I am trying to suppress the unpleasant nausea that follows. My chest begins to feel like it itches from the inside, and it is heavy. Ugh. It is so heavy. Like I cannot take a deep breath. In fact, I cannot breathe at all. My arms and legs become heavier than lead weights. They want to move me, but I cannot seem to connect my brain to my extremities, and so I am frozen in place. I feel the urge to open my mouth, but nothing comes out. I do not even think my lips part. My mood becomes somber, and I just get this overall feeling of dread. The only thing that seems doable is finding somewhere to lie down and hide.

Usually, I want to go to my room and be alone, but I do not want anyone to know that I am there or that I am falling apart—and yet, at the same time, I crave another human's presence to hold me and tell me I am safe and it is all okay. Usually, that other human I crave is my husband, and usually he does not know that I'm breaking. Hello, shame. And, side note: that is as intimate as I will ever get about my marriage on this (*or any*) platform.

I just end up sitting wherever I landed. Feeling completely and absolutely fucked because there is nowhere to go and no one to turn to. If I am being honest, I think I dissociate from where I am. I feel like I have left my body and my reality, and I curse myself for reacting this way.

My mind is transported back to a fight or flight response, but apparently my limbic system does a *"shut down and freak the fuck out"* instead of anything helpful. Once I am triggered, I have these feelings for anywhere from minutes to hours to days. My mind cannot let go and my body cannot move.

It is pretty unpleasant.

I have been in counseling for a couple decades, and while I have narrowed my triggers down from about twenty different things to three, when one or all of the three sneak up uninvited, it is overwhelming.

Before I knew what was happening, before I recognized this as a trigger response, it terrified the living shit out of me. When you spend all your time repressing shit and then all of a sudden, out of nowhere, in the least convenient place, it all comes flooding back and taking you along, it tends to send a chill down your spine.

I was just reading. I was not expecting to be thrown into the middle of an anxious meltdown. It is not how I planned to spend my week.

The book had no trigger warnings. There were no hints that this was coming until I was already reading it, and then my eyes could not turn away because I was frozen. But they could still move through the words, and my brain could still comprehend. And it hurt to read, but I read it. So why am I telling you this?

Because maybe you know someone with PTSD. And maybe you have seen them be fine one second and then the next moment they have left you behind. And maybe they cannot tell you where they are or what they need.

Maybe they do not even know.

And maybe you find yourself taking it personally. Like you have done something wrong. Like they have left *you*. And I can only imagine over time how that wears down a person who loves someone with PTSD. So I wanted to tell you where we go. We slip back into whatever hellish trauma we have survived, and we are paralyzed by it. We are at its mercy, and all we can do is wait for it to pass.

My counselor has tried to give me coping skills to handle these situations. Like to tell myself that I am safe, and it is not really happening again—but it just does not seem to help.

The truth is I fight every day to feel any sense of security, and when I am triggered it reminds me how very fragile the feeling of safety actually is. How very fragile *being safe* is.

I wish I could tell you how to best support someone who has PTSD, but I do not think I can. I think that the support needed might depend on the person.

In my case, I do not want to talk about it. I already cannot find my voice, and it does not feel safe to use it. I do not want to explain myself, and I do not want to comfort the person who feels alienated by my involuntary visitation to the painful realm of trauma.

But it is nice to have someone sit with me. Without saying a word. Without adding any extra burden to my already over-burdened mind.

I found myself unexpectedly triggered and without the words to communicate that to my people, and I thought maybe other warriors feel the same. While this should not be considered a guide for how to help someone struggling with PTSD, maybe it can serve as a starting point for how you can help them without putting extra pressure on their already over-worked system.

Maybe you can just sit with them. Letting them know you are there, and they are safe.

And maybe one day they will believe you enough to tell you where they go when they leave, and how you can help them find their way back to you and their ever-elusive safe space.

LOVE, DEPRESSION

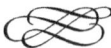

I had a moment this morning on my way to work. I was driving along a country highway with my windows rolled down, absorbing the chill in the air. I noticed the trees along the roadway and wondered if they were actually turning colors or if they always had streaks of banana-yellow and rust-red in them.

It is funny because I drive down that road every damn day, and I have no idea what color the trees usually are. Either I am the world's most oblivious human or the absolutely most focused driver, and let us just say, it ain't the latter.

Anyway.

The sky was as clear as blue glass, and the sun shining on the center of my forehead might have blinded my eyes, had I been just one inch taller. I am not going to lie, I had my minivan stereo turned up embarrassingly loud and was belting out the words to my new favorite song, and all of a sudden I thought to myself:

"Woah. I am not depressed today."

If I am being honest, that is the first time I have been able to mean those words in forty-two days.

I know.

I talk a lot about coping mechanisms and managing mental health and chasing joy and all the things in that wheelhouse, and still it found me. This is usually the point where I get a lot of:

"No ways" and *"I had no ideas"* and *"Why didn't you say anythings?"*

I think the short answer to those questions is that I did not want to.

I did not want to talk about it, and I did not want anyone to know. I mean, I never do. Why burden people with my stuff when they are going through their own? So I just chug along, internally deteriorating and giving the outward illusion that I am maintaining mental wellness. It is exhausting and, honestly, not what I would recommend. Especially now that I feel better, you better believe that I am a *"tell someone when you are struggling because you matter and they care"* advocate. And I mean that wholeheartedly.

But I often do not afford myself that same grace. I am sure many of us battling depression do not. I *did* contemplate writing about how it actually felt to be experiencing depression —or, more accurately, the lack of feelings that depression brings. Like an actual play-by-play, real-time account of a depressive episode; but that was a bummer (even to me), and I honestly think that it can be triggering.

So I cowered away in isolation whenever I could. If I did not have to be on, let me tell you, I was off.

Generally speaking, the people who only see you when you are 'on' will never know. And that is by design. But you can only hide it from the person you fall asleep and wake up next to for so long. There were plenty of *"Are you okay?"* and *"You seem a little depressed?"* questions being asked from said bed partner.

And they were all met with no eye contact, teeth covered, half smiles *"I'm fine"* responses. Until finally I decided it was pointless to try and hide what was happening from the man who changed my last name. I must say that my husband is an actual saint for sticking by me despite this mental illness thing. Ugh. Even I hate the words mental illness. Even I feel the stigma of them judging me harshly.

Anyway.

I often wonder: if the roles were reversed, would I be able to do it? Would I be able to handle the days upon days of withdrawal. The insecurities. The incessant sadness. Without absorbing it. And becoming it? Maybe we do not pull at that thread?

Anyway.

Rest assured, I am better. In fact, that is the only reason I am showing up here now. Even though depression tells me that I am all alone and no one has ever felt as nothing as I feel, I know that I am not the only one battling this disease. The one that tells us all the lies and makes it so easy for us to succumb to them.

Now, here is the thing. Everyone always wants to know *"why you are depressed"* because, well, depression is for people who have shitty circumstances and make awful life choices.

Nurp.

The most concise answer I can formulate is that depression is a chronic illness. One that I must work to manage. However, sometimes it flares up. Sometimes it flares up because I forgot to take my medication regularly and sometimes it flares up because I have a PTSD moment and—despite my best efforts

—I just cannot seem to navigate my way out of the black hole that is eating me alive. And sometimes I think it just flares up for its own amusement.

This might be where you think that I should be utilizing all the coping mechanisms in my metaphorical toolbox, but not so much.

Not only does depression hijack your mind, but it also takes your energy. Who has the energy to do things when all your body seems to be capable of is rest?

Luckily, I *did* go to counseling amid all of this. I do not always come out feeling better, but I almost always come out with a better understanding of what is happening inside this poorly wired brain of mine. And also, I sometimes kid because being serious for too long makes me wildly uncomfortable.

Anyway.

I cannot be the only one who feels like there is this overall *"get over it"* attitude when a person is struggling with their mental health. I think it is generally expected that our mood is within our control, so we should be able to 'gratitude-journal' our way out of depression. And if we do not, then we are choosing it.

All I can say to that is: suicide is the tenth leading cause of death in the United States. Depression is an actual illness in which people find themselves fighting for their life. Like other disease processes, sometimes they lose that battle. I think that maybe with a little more compassion and awareness and a little less shame and guilt, we can change those statistics for the better.

Anyway.

I was probably three weeks into this mental illness nightmare before I realized what was happening. I do not know where the lightbulb moment came from because it certainly was not my head. I think it was my gut. In my gut I knew something was not right. I have been battling depression for over twenty-five years, and I still find it difficult to recognize when it exacerbates.

Anyway.

That brings us to this day. I was listening to "You are going to be Ok" by Jenn Johnson for the 300-millionth time because it inadvertently became my theme song when Spotify peered into my soul and added it to my recommended songs list. It hit me like a Santa sack of glitter and hope that I had gotten through it. I made it to the other side, and I just want to say that this side is lighter and brighter and, simply, better.

Anyway.

I just wanted to tell you that I spent six weeks in the trenches, waiting for the fog to lift and beginning to think that it never would. I abandoned all coping mechanisms, and people that I did not have to see. I spent more time hiding under blankets, trying to cover tears, than I care to admit. And then I woke up today, when nothing had changed, but everything was different.

The ultimate point here, my beautiful warrior friends, is this: it *will* pass. It *will* get better. Keep going. And when you feel like depression has stolen the goodness that is your coping mechanisms, your medication benefits, and your life-giving mantras, then I have two suggestions:

1. Talk to your person—whoever that is—and ask them if you can be 'off' with them. FYI: they will say yes.

2. Find yourself a song that you can blast on repeat until the fog lifts.

You will feel something again, and let me tell you, that something is worth it.

INKLINGS

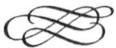

" **B** *iblical hope and practical help.*"
I read that on the back of a pocket-sized devotional my counselor recommended, and if it's not completely powerful, then I do not know what is. I feel like it summarizes my mental health journey so beautifully.

"Biblical hope and practical help."

Ugh, so good.

My whole mental wellness endeavor has been one of trying to coordinate mind, body, and spirit into explicit harmony. I am going to chat about something that has truly helped me: tattoos.

Let us chat ink therapy.

Now, I think I am pretty much officially considered middle-aged; like on the older end of the mid-life spectrum. I may even have had a midlife crisis *(or three)*. I know I get sidetracked easily, but talking about how old I am *is* pertinent to this story, and here is why.

I grew up in a time where tattoos were saddled with the stigma of being trashy and unprofessional. A sign flashing that you are of a low socioeconomic status. On the flip side, they cost a small fortune, so make that make sense.

It is so deeply ingrained in me that if you are of the 60+ community, I pretty much try to hide what I have etched on my skin at all costs. Because y'all, as a generalized whole, still try and look down on recreationally tattooed people. And because I am semi politically correct, I will add an "in my experience" so as not to offend any boomers.

I never seem to have the emotional energy to explain why I, a middle-aged mother of five, is suddenly tatted up. Until now that is.

I am really into words (*if you have not noticed*) and symbolism (*if that was not obvious*) and, in my opinion, tattoos offer both.

When I was going through my suicidal ideation, I made a promise to my husband that I would not go through with it. As a person who values words, that promise might as well have been its own form of red words—and if you know the Bible, you know that the "red words" are the words of Jesus. The problem with that was I did not really think myself capable of keeping said promise. So I did what any symbolist would do, and I started desperately looking for anything that made it more bearable. Somehow, I landed on a tattoo. Permanently placing a promise on your body is the ultimate symbol of words mattering.

If you are a Gen X'er or older, then you are probably *thinking just write it down on, like, a piece of paper.* Or actually open your Bible and find solace there. Okay, I hear you—but, also, I have a drawer full of quote books and notebooks and journals and less than stellar self-help masterpieces with all the reminders and techniques for how to live your best life. Yet when I am in the middle of a nervous breakdown, the last thing on my mind is which book had that one thing that will help me out of that particular headspace.

Turns out the whole process was wildly therapeutic. Every time I was unsure I had it in me to keep that promise, I would look in the mirror at my hidden reminder and somehow tap into an internal strength I did not know I had.

I have since gotten five more to equal three tattoos. I know I am awful at math, but this equation will add up. You will see. It makes me a little cringey to break out the visual and meanings of said art, but somehow this seems like as good a place as any to step outside that comfort zone and do it anyway. Do not try to understand my brain. It is un-understandable.

Here is what I got.

A sign of my lasting obsession with the healing properties of lavender-laden aromatherapy and the healing magic of breath work. It is near my wrist, and therefore it is incredibly easy for me to simply glance down in the middle of an excruciatingly busy or painful day and pause for deep breaths.

And if I can, spritz the ish out of myself with lavender oil.

Next up is a beauty that I utilize even more. It is on my inner-upper arm: a namaste yoga silhouette intertwined with a hummingbird and the words *"Keep going."*

I cannot tell you the number of times I have found myself wanting to quit. Doing the work is so hard, but it is also so worth it. And that is what that one means to me. It reminds me that no matter how many backward steps I take, I can still pick myself back up and move forward. (*Clever hummingbird reference, eh?*)

And of course, when in doubt, bust the mat out of some yoga.

Last but not least, there is a three-in-one one. I mentioned it earlier and it is by far the most personal and vulnerable art I have. That is why I have it on my back—so I can easily tuck it away from the world.

Hi, stigma. Howdy, shame. How y'all doin'?

That is the one that started it all. I have been adding to it over the last three years. It started with the semicolon and birds; that was my promise tattoo.

Then I went through my IOP program and knew that I was not still around only because I promised to be, but because I *wanted* to be and that was so powerful that I needed to immortalize it. So I had the dandelion added, you know in relation to mental health and perspective. To be honest, I thought that one was done. I had come full circle, literally, and it (*and I*) felt complete. But life keeps happening—as it must—and I realized that I cannot fit my journey into a perfect circle, nor is said journey complete. After all, I am still alive (*and grateful to be*). I recently, as in last week, had five more dandelion seeds and even more birds and yet another word in the form of 'trust' added. If that is not a loaded masterpiece, then I do not know what is.

My sister asked me if it was complete now, and I told her that my story is not over yet, so no. No, it is not. I do not know the next chapter of my story, but this tattoo will eventually tell it. Okay. That was my long-winded way of saying that I have found hope and healing and meaning and purpose in tattoos.

Let me go ahead and do the responsible writer thing and say this:

You should not go get a tattoo just because I (*or anyone, for that matter*) find it therapeutic. Permanent changes to your person cannot be taken lightly. Marinade on the idea for a lot longer than you think you need to. And picture it on your skin for for.ev.er. Imagine it hanging out on your fine self on the day where you meet royalty and have on a gussied-up lace gown and fancy hairdo. See if you mind having it in the midst of all that, and then you can start your personal transformation with a less committal form of change with, like, a haircut. And then venture into some hair dye, and so on and so forth.

Finding *your* joy is deeply personal. It is also deeply necessary. No one can tell you what will heal you, except you. But when you find it, unapologetically consume it. And forget all the haters (*to prove I am still young enough to use a millennial colloquialism*) who think you should curate yourself differently.

Unless it is yoga. Then trust. That will heal the ish outta ya.

THE CASE FOR YOGA

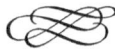

I am a yoga fanatic. Not to be dramatic or anything, but it has changed my life. Whenever someone starts to talk to me about anxiety or stress, or really anything, I am all like, *"But have you tried yoga?"*

Remember *My Big Fat Greek Wedding* where Tula's dad's magic cure for everything was Windex?

That is me, except my Windex is yoga.

I have not studied yoga per se or its origin story. However, I have been coming to my mat long enough that wanting to know the ins and outs of it all is now on my bucket list. I am mentioning this because every year that I can remember, *Yoga with Adriene (who I find somewhat of an inspiration, but also read: I am an absolute fan girl)* starts the New Year off with a 30-day Yoga Journey. And every year, I start it with her. And every year for the past, oh I do not know, three to five years, I have completed, like, fifteen days.

Which usually takes me twenty-seven days just to get in fifteen days. And then I am done because if we are going to be technical about it, I did thirty days of yoga. The "daily" part is a minor detail.

But one year I was determined to do thirty daily days of yoga, and if you cannot sense the faux confidence in my words, just know that by day two I was already doubting my ability to succeed.

Why did I suddenly become determined to complete a full-on yoga challenge? Because I was curious.

I wanted to know what was going to happen if I showed up to my mat every single day for thirty straight days.

What would happen physically and mentally and emotionally and spiritually and all the -ally ways.

What would discipline and consistency teach me?

Would my anxiety be better controlled? Because, y'all: real talk. At times, a lot of times, the anxiety threatens to swallow me whole. In those moments, I not only reach into my toolbox for all the coping mechanisms, but I also cling to them tightly.

Yoga is one of those mechanisms. It has helped manage my mental illness so beautifully that it would be a betrayal of self if I did not actually make the time to do this.

You know what else yoga compliments so wonderfully? Jesus. When you are deep in breath and meditation, it is a beautiful moment to invite prayer. And I wanted to say that because I know that there are a lot of people who think that mental illness can be managed by God and are probably shouting to these pages, *"Have you opened your Bible to help with your anxiety?"* and the answer is yes. And the honest answer is not nearly enough, but in addition to showing up consistently on my mat, I am working on showing up consistently in my faith.

If I have to rate the tools in my toolbox, I am clinging to Jesus first and yoga second.

When it comes to implementing the elements of our toolboxes, it feels like the results are out of our control. Whether it is sick kids or soul-sucking post-pandemic days that leave us too exhausted to do anything else, it feels like our circumstances are in control of our actions.

And maybe they are.

But that kind of thinking makes my anxiety go through the roof. As an anxious person, I must find and root myself in what I can control.

So, I have to remember that unexpected and undesirable events will always be happening around me. The roadblocks are real. But how I respond *is* within my control, and doing the things that keep me going...

... I *do* have control over that.

Therefore, I finished the challenge, nay, journey with a plan. I did not think about Day 30. I thought about Day 1 on Day 1, and Day 2 on Day 2, and so on and so forth. And on that day, I committed to a time when I could be on my mat, and each day the time was different. I just need to continue to live in the present and remind myself (*constantly*) that I am worthy of doing the things that make me a better human.

And so are you. In case you ever doubted it.

And if that is not the definition of practice, then I do not know what is.

I truly cannot help myself when it comes to thinking about yoga and talking about yoga and thinking about talking about yoga because it is just so good. I mean life changing-ly good.

Like I said, I have been wanting to delve further into yoga. Like really dive into the roots and origins of the practice and the scientifically proven health benefits of the practice (*because let me tell you that based on personal experience, I know the health benefits of yoga*). And I want to hear (*hello, podcasts*) and read what actual yoga gurus have to say on the matter.

And I was thinking how when I tell someone about yoga and how yummy it is and they are all like, "*Yoga isn't my thing,*" and I'm all like, "*I'm sorry, I don't understand what you just said,*" that it has taken me a minute to get borderline obsessed with yoga. I did not just wake up one day and suddenly want to be a yoga expert. It has been ten years since I first discovered the practice and, what the heck, let us do an "*It all started when*"... segment.

It all started when...

I birthed my second child and my postpartum hormones somehow started settling down, I began to think outside of my own anxieties. I wanted to get back in shape—flat tummy and pre-pregnancy clothes—because then my goals were different. I had done the conventional gym membership/ personal trainer after my first pregnancy, and I hated every second of it. Actually, I had a buddy to go with, so that part was fun, but I did not find joy in the work out. I knew that returning to "*working out*" to get in shape was not what I wanted. But I still had a gym membership, and lo and behold, they offered some combination classes of yoga and Pilates, and I think they called it Pi-Yo.

I fell in love.

I looked forward to my weekly time-away-from-my-responsibilities classes because it was time for myself that I truly enjoyed. I tapped into something that I think I lost when I became a mother knee-deep in babies and toddlers. I know you are not supposed to say this, but I am saying it anyway.

We lose ourselves in motherhood, and there is no reward for doing so. In fact, I think the best thing we can do for our kids is to maintain our frailties. We did not become superhuman when we became moms, so why do all signs of the world say we should act like it?

As we all know, gym memberships and exercise-class costs become onerous and can seem frivolous. So when something has to get removed from the budget, we get rid of the things we think are extras—and my soul-reviving Pi-Yo was one of them. This was before I realized the importance of self-care and how it impacted my spirit. This was also before the time of free YouTube (*or at least I had no knowledge of it if it was available*), and we still had to spend money on workout videos.

Y'all, I may as well be ancient.

I remember trying to find a free and affordable place where I could jump back into the realm of yoga because I knew what it was doing for me. It took me another five years of dabbling in the idea of yoga before I discovered Adriene for freezies *(do we say things like freezies anymore?)* on YouTube, and *BAM*.

My perfect workout scenario: free yoga at home. Like, I did not have to talk to people.

Not to be antisocial, but that is definitely my jam.

Anyhoo *(do we still say anyhoo?)*, I fell in love with Adriene. Obviously, everyone has considering her 10 million subscribers on YouTube. The woman is a force to reckon with. The thing that I respect the most about her is that if you watch her older videos and compared to now, she is literally the same. Same vibe and still humble. And one day, when I am rich and famous, I vow to stay the same.

I mean, if I am going to go for it, I may as well *go* for it.

Also, I am kidding. I have no desire to remain humble.

Kidding.

Anyway, I did online Adriene yoga for a while and then felt this nagging need to escalate my yoga practice. I heard about this thing called hot yoga. I hate sweating, so I was semi skeptical, and in fact had asked myself a few times, "*What kind of psycho would do hot yoga?*"

It's me.

Somehow, I got conned into going and surprisingly, it was the best thing ever. I converted. There is something about the ice cold, essential-oil-clad cloth at the end of practice that made sweating worth it. I went once a week until COVID, and then, you know, I lost my mojo.

To be fair, I think we all did.

I have since rediscovered the joys of home practice and incorporating daily yoga into my routine, and the more I practice the more I am convinced that yoga will save humanity.

Now, do not get your panties in a bunch. I know that Jesus saves humanity. But I think we can have Jesus AND yoga.

I get that it is not everyone's cup of tea, and to that I say: *but it is.* You just do not know it yet.

Yoga brings self-awareness, mindfulness, and intention into my day to day. It also helps to deepen my faith and desire to know my Savior. I am literally a calmer and kinder human being when I start and end my day with yoga. It has taught me that I am worthy of slowing down. That I am worthy of taking time.

That I am worth being better.

It has let me be unapologetically big and loud and unafraid to take up as much space as I can possibly take. I am more motivated to continue on the path of self-improvement, and I am so convicted on consistency I can hardly stand it.

To sum up: everything is better.

And when I look at our world and what is happening in it, don't we all just want better?

MEDICATION CONFESSIONAL

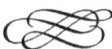

You know I may (or may not) have mentioned once or twice that I take medications for my anxiety and depression. As such, sometimes I think that if we were to find ourselves in a zombie apocalypse (*because all rational thoughts start with 'zombie apocalypse'*) that my mental health would take a hit when I ran out of medication.

How am I supposed to survive the stress of a post-apocalyptic world without pharmaceutical intervention?

I probably spend more time thinking about this than I should. But, alas, I have not been able to come up with a solution, strategy, or plan for the above scenario should it occur.

And that deeply concerns me.

Should I be more concerned about the fact that I am spending time and energy mulling on less than likely end-of-the-world scenarios?

Possibly. But to use another popular bit of terminology: it is what it is.

What ends up happening is that I find myself feeling weak because I need medication to survive.

I know. But sometimes I think I have something to prove. I think that I should not have to rely on artificial neurotransmitters to keep my brain whole.

I do not know who I think I have to *"prove anything"* to...

To myself?

To the world?

Still working that one out.

But I figure if I think it, then someone else probably does too. And I wanted to share how I keep going when the guilt and shame of treatment infiltrate my mental-health-matters armor.

Without medication, I have not been able to navigate my mental illness. No, that is a lie. I have navigated it but not well, and not in a manner that I would recommend to anyone. My coping mechanisms are less than stellar when I am not on medicine. The thing about it is I have tried to come off the antidepressants and the medications that help manage my physical manifestations of anxiety. Especially when I start to feel well.

I think to myself, *"I bet I could do this without medicine,"* and, *"I'm stronger than depression."*

As if sheer willpower will change or supplement the chemicals in my brain.

If I said I did not at times wish to keep on keeping on without the need for medication, I would be lying. Y'all know I journal and I do yoga and intuitive eating, and all the things that are supposed to manage anxiety and depression, but here is the thing: those things do not manage brain chemicals.

They do not keep me on an even playing ground.

It gets tricky talking about medicine and mental illness because even though there are your basic combinations and first-line prescriptions, the way they react within everyone is unique, and my experience with specific medications may not be your experience.

Which is why I do not usually name which medications I am on, or which did or did not work for me. I think it would be irresponsible, and that is a conversation that should happen between a provider and a patient, not through a one-sided conversation on a page.

However, here's one thing that I do believe helped me find the right combination of medications after a lot of trial and error: genetic testing. And I have two disclaimers:

1. *Always* talk to your healthcare provider to determine the best course of action for your specific situation;
2. Letting you know that this testing helped me and my doctor find the right medications for me (*notice all the Me's I am using*) is *not* me offering medical advice. It is simply me sharing my experience.

Now that we have that out of the way, back to my anecdotal story.

I also sometimes find myself wondering: if "so and so" knew I had to take medicine to function, they would think less of me.

Who is '*so and so*'?

No idea. I think it is some faux imaginative beings that my subconscious fabricates. They have no name and no face, and they are judging me harshly in the zombie apocalypse.

And I guess the next question that lingers in my brain is:

What do I mean when I say, *"I need medication to function?"*

Well, let me tell you that when I am not on medication, my

depression ravages my brain. It incapacitates me. My thoughts go from not helpful to deeply self-mutilating. And I cannot control them or the nothingness. I fade into this black hole in which the despair is so deep there is no climbing out. Essentially, I am the pages 22-42 of this book.

Medicine keeps me on this side of despair. The side that allows me to go to work. Raise my kids. Communicate in my marriage. Get out of bed in the mornings. Take a shower. Write. Yoga. It keeps me from suffocating in the darkness.

Most days I am grateful that medication for mental illness exists. That there are people standing against the dangerous stigma associated with asking for help.

But that stigma is still somehow buried deep within me because I feel unsure about writing this book.

So here is what I tell myself when the self-sabotaging thoughts creep in.

I remember that it is *not* my fault that I have a mental illness. Depression and anxiety are *not* choices I make. They are *not* feelings. They *are* diagnoses. They are actual illnesses that require actual medical intervention.

I remind myself that taking medication is *not a weakness*. In fact, it is a strength. To realize that you need help and then to go after help and then to accept help and then to be consistent with treatment requires some major internal motivation and strength.

And, lastly, I tell myself that in the event of a zombie apocalypse, I am scrappy enough to wade through pharmacies and get my refills.

TILL HYGIENE PARTS US

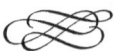

My experience with depression is not sadness. In fact, I do not feel sad at all.

I just do not feel.

There may be uncontrollable sobbing, loss of interest in things I once enjoyed, lack of motivation, finding it difficult to get going in the morning—or any time of day, really. An inability to sleep through the night. But mostly it is numbness.

The biggest IDGAF because I feel nothing.

This may be a taboo subject, but that signals to me that I should write about it. As I have mentioned before, my writings are not about a unique individual who has unusual experiences. It is about the average Jane muddling through life. I am willing to bet that there is another soul out there who can relate to what I am going to say.

So, here we go.

In 2019, I turned our world upside down when I revealed to my husband that I was suicidal.

By doing so, I opened a delicate door that I had been holding shut with all my might for ten years.

Picture *Game of Thrones* Hodor here.

The struggle has been real. I have been on a journey of learning to manage my depression rather than pushing it down to the deepest part of my stomach only for it to come out to play with a vengeance later.

For me, managing depression means being aware of when I am slipping down that unpleasant rabbit hole. Throughout the course of my treatment and with the power of hindsight, I learned that there were a lot, tons if you will, of red flags signaling that my depression was poorly managed. I made a mental note to deal with it later—because who has time now?

One of those signs was hygiene.

Insert *'ew'* here.

However, I was unaware of the connection between showering and depression. And I should go ahead and insert a mind-blown emoji to symbolize the impact this realization has had on me.

I was asked several times during my intake interview how often I showered. My reply was,

"Whenever I need to."

That was an honest answer. And isn't that when everyone showers?

But apparently the definition of 'my needing to' and of a 'healthy need to' were different.

Mindfulness matters, folks.

As I went through the program, I was asked every session about my bathing habits. I also listened to others discuss theirs. And I realized: I had stopped caring. I could go days without turning on water thanks to dry shampoo and deodorant.

I really do not know if anyone noticed; no one said anything to me. Other than my husband.

Hi, hindsight.

Looking back, my husband would ask me:

"Did you shower today?"

And I would give him an evil stare, taking complete offense. Not realizing he was checking in on my mental health.

I came to realize that I was not showering on the regular because there was no point in doing so, says depression.

So now, I check in with myself.

Has it been a minute since I showered?

Is it because I am a working mom of five and ran out of time?

Or is it because taking care of myself is pointless?

Either way, I hop in the shower.

You can insert a sigh of relief here.

But, if the answer is the latter, I have then made myself aware that my depression is taking hold, and I need to be extra diligent in implementing my coping mechanisms.

I find depression to be a chronic illness. One that I am doing my best to manage. One that I *have to do the things* to manage it.

It is hard when it is your mind that is sick; after all, when it is a physical illness people say:

"Keep a positive attitude," and,

"Look at the bright side."

Insinuating that the path to wellness is mind over matter.

I have always struggled with how to do that when it is my mind that hurts.

I guess I just must tell myself to keep going.

And hope that it works.

So far, so good.

THRIVE IN THERAPY

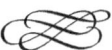

Currently, I am improving, I am more than improving, I think I can say that I am, in fact, thriving.

But if I am being a hundred percent honest, then I must also admit that I am terrified. I no longer have suicidal ideation, but at times I am filled with overwhelming fear. The truth is that I may have won the battle, but the war rages on. Mental illness is not a sprint to the finish line. You do not get to a certain point and conquer it—you learn how to manage it. It is an ongoing journey of self-discovery. Of learning what works and what does not. Of falling off the proverbial horse and getting back on. In short, it is exhausting.

Putting my battles out into the world provokes a certain fear. I cannot tell you the number of mental blocks I have come across when writing these pages. So many of them are this voice shouting, "No one cares!"

And maybe that is true.

I fear facing those who only know me on the surface to acknowledge that I have been struggling because they probably do not care.

Or maybe that is the mental illness telling me that. Or the devil. Poe-tae-toh, Poe-tah-toe.

Either way, it is scary to face those who thought I had it all together and was managing just fine and acknowledging that, in fact, I was not. I am also scared of saying I am better because then everyone expects that I am okay.

I do not see how I will ever be the same. I was lost in a black hole for so long, desperately reaching toward the surface, that now that I can breathe, I like it.

The view is different up here.

But it.is.work.

However, so is struggling. If these pages have imparted anything, it should be that ignoring the problem only helps for so long—and in the end, it does not help at all.

I still need medication and yoga. And let us not forget Jesus. But I also need counseling.

Regularly.

I need coping mechanisms.

Something that we do not talk about often is how hard therapy is because, God, it can be hard. Working through trauma will gut you and challenge you and leave you questioning if healing is not just impossible but if it is actually worth it.

I always liken therapy days to peeling the layers of an onion. I realize that I have only just begun paring away layers and there is oh-so-much-more to peel to get to the core—and much like peeling an onion, there will almost always be tears involved.

What I bring into my therapist's office is rarely what I leave it with, which is always a deeper understanding of what is contributing to my mental load.

As someone who is on the never-ending rollercoaster of

understanding how trauma has interwoven itself into every facet of her mental illness and also her life, and as someone who is constantly working on healing from the consequences of trauma, I just want to tell you it is worth it.

You probably want to know why and how and what makes it worth it, and all I can say is that there is something about learning that you are worthy and lovable and loved that will lighten your chest and relax your muscles and free up space in your mind and send your spirit soaring in gratitude and increase your capacity to pour into others—because you aren't using all of your precious energy to hold on to a pain that you didn't ask to endure.

So, yes, keep peeling the layers even when your eyes are blinded by the burning because one day you will wake up and realize that what you thought made you broken actually makes you beautiful.

Living a life free from the chains of unprocessed trauma is truly a life worth living.

PART II

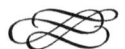

PART II
FAIRY-TALE FODDER

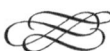

There is no doubt that living with mental illness is hard. However, I can only imagine how hard it is to be married to someone with depression. Or how difficult it is to be raised by a mom who has a hard enough time navigating her own emotions, let alone teaching her children how to navigate theirs.

It is me. I am someone.

Someone's wife, someone's mother. Just out here, constantly breaking down and falling short and simultaneously asking for forgiveness and welcoming grace.

I sometimes say to my husband: "Lance, do you really love me?"

And he will say, "Of course I do."

And I remain unconvinced, and I can see the discouragement in my husband's eyes because he knows there is nothing he can say that will make me believe him. It is up to me to find my own value and believe in my own worth.

And then there are times where my son will say to me: "Mom, do you really love me?"

And I will say, "Of course I do." And I'll add a "more than anything" to really drive the point home.

And I can see it in his eyes that he remains undecided if my words ring true, and it is a reminder that I cannot control my son's anxiety, but I can teach him how to manage it. If there is only one thing I get right in this life, I want it to be that.

The following essays, therefore, are meant to highlight how depression and anxiety can infiltrate marriage and mother-hood, and also how mental wellness can restore what mental illness will not stop trying to steal.

I think that the biggest takeaway I hope to leave you with after you read the following chapters is this:

Your "as is" self is beautiful.

And that is the self that your people want.

At the end of the day,

Your people want to help you be okay.

Your people want to help you.

Your people want you.

RELATIONSHIP EVOLUTION

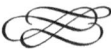

"What was your last name?" my son curiously asks.

"Before I met daddy? Kur-ray-bet. Until I got married. Now it is the same as yours."

"So is your mom's name Khuraibet?" he concludes.

"Well, it used to be. Not anymore though. Momma's parents aren't married anymore."

"I know. That is sad. He's a good grandpa."

"It makes me sad too. But I suppose just because someone is a good grandpa, doesn't mean they are a good husband."

"Mmmm."

I see him absorbing the heavy words.

"That is big, tough stuff, bud. Only they know why they aren't married."

"Yeah."

I met my husband when I was eighteen. My parents divorced when I was twenty-nine. The reason that their marriage fell apart after thirty-three years is still hard for me to comprehend. But that is not my story to tell; it is theirs.

What is mine to tell, however, is the effect that their relationship and subsequent divorce has on a grown child with an eventual family of her own. I did not know the extent of the pain until I started peeling layers and wondering why the idea of marriage, to me, was disposable.

Grief is not limited to death. It applies to any situation where something of significance has ended and, for me, my parents' marriage ending was significant.

Growing up, I found their relationship to be one of chatter and laughter. They would spend car rides discussing their current circumstances and plans for the future. I always admired that. I remember them holding hands while talking and thinking, "I hope to have that one day."

They also laughed, a lot. My dad would make my mom give the largest belly laugh I had ever heard on numerous occasions, and hearing her laugh and laughing myself brought me relief. A sense of happiness and joy that I otherwise never felt. It was during those times that I learned the healing power of humor and decided to find more of it. Did my childhood beer goggles romanticize things a bit? Perhaps. But isn't that the magic of childhood that we so desperately try to preserve? Seeing the good in people and believing that even the most complicated pains have a simple fix?

Needless to say, when I met my husband I was looking for someone I could talk to, and someone who would make me laugh. And, boy, did he deliver; the man is hysterical. He makes me laugh harder than I ever thought was possible. That laughter brings me emotional release and peace of mind, and I appreciate him for it. In fact, the moment we met is engrained into my brain, and often when I look at him today, I flash back to when I first saw him. That man is my dream come true. I remember walking into a room where he was strumming an acoustic guitar, his back to me and all I could see was his perfect nose, milk-chocolate-brown hair, strong hands and manly build, with a burning cigarette loosely hanging out the side of his mouth. He turned around to acknowledge my entrance, and then I saw his ocean-colored eyes and I fell into a feeling I had never known. He is, in fact, the love of my life. Not that I go around broadcasting it to him. He is probably as shocked at reading this as I am at admitting it, but every once in a while I let it slip.

But we did not get to a place of laughter and mutual unspoken understanding overnight. In fact, it has taken years of love, sweat, and tears. Fights that I figured would break us because their intensity seemed unforgivable. Sometimes I wonder how we made it. To be honest, if it were all up to me, we would not have. I did not know that marriage was sacred. I did not know that people worked through their problems. I did not know that love could grow through trials and tribulations. And before you go thinking, "Well, that's because you're a child of divorce," I was not. My parents were married my entire childhood. It is interesting how a person forms ideas regardless of their environment. The only plausible reason I can come up with for my belief that marriage was disposable is that I must have been divorced in another life. Which is to say, I do not have any plausible reason for why it took me eight years to take my vows seriously.

My husband has always honored a "I will love you through this because I married you and that means something" promise. A love that I did not know existed. I never really believed that men loved people. I am sure there is a lot we can unpack there, like all the self-hate I harbored, but for now I am going to leave that unpacking within the walls of my therapist's office.

The evolution in our relationship consisted of me bleeding

my unhealed trauma all over him and him choosing to help me heal. I do not know what I did to deserve it, but our marriage has absolutely been the catalyst and reason for my growth and healing. I am truly a better person for having found him, and I am so grateful he did not give up on me.

Before anyone gets their pants in a tizzy, I am not advocating anyone should stay in toxic, unhealthy, or abusive relationships. But if your person is broken and wants to heal, and you have the capacity to hold him or her through it, you deserve gratitude.

They say the first year of marriage is rough, and I would like to build upon that notion and let you know that the first eight years of marriage are rough. And then, it is still rough, but somewhere along the line, if you keep going you will learn the beauty of communication and the power in it. You will learn what it really means to love. You will learn that the fights were really just fears and you faced them together and are stronger for it. You will learn things about yourself you did not know. For example, I did not trust my husband.

Now, of course I thought I did. When I was point-blank asked whether or not I trusted my husband, I was offended and defensive and would return the question with an adamant answer of, "It's not about trust."

Huh? I guess you can call that an answer if you want. Truthfully, it is only now in reflection and counseling that I have been able to both learn and admit that I, in fact, did not.

A lot of things happen in a year. And many more happen in a decade or two. We had babies, we lost jobs, we lost money, we lost faith. There have been funerals and goodbyes to family members that were not quite as final as death but have still led to quite a bit of grief.

I think the most unsettling part of a divorce you do not see coming is that it begs the question: what cracks are in our marriage that I am not seeing? Which ones will rear their ugly head twenty-five years down the road? Especially when you happen upon an anniversary card that your mom wrote to your dad: "Happy anniversary. Thank you for twenty-one years of happiness." And you wonder at what point that stopped being true.

I have no idea what the future holds for my marriage, but isn't that true of all futures? All I know is that we have been together for twenty-one years, and I think our story is just getting started.

BREAKING POINT

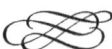

I do not know if I can accurately describe how a mental breakdown feels. I stopped making decisions. I handed that responsibility over to my husband the moment I realized what was happening, and to be honest I have not been too keen to take that responsibility back. When I finally acknowledged to myself that I would end my life and then subsequently admitted that to my husband, he told me I had to get help. Which means I had to tell people. And that realization takes you from entering a mental breakdown into having a full-fledged one. All the energy that I had put into holding on to everything I was feeling and experiencing leached out of my skin and went into the room around me. I guess you could say it was freeing. The sobs that followed my confession were guttural and primal. I had no control over their release, and I certainly did not have the strength to stop them.

"I-deep breath-just-sob-don't want-sob-people to-whimper-sob-know."

The thought of telling people that I was broken was too much to bear, and figuring out how to put myself back together was impossible. So I guess I learned about my first boundary in the moment—and my limits. I could not do it. I handed the responsibility off to him, and I am eternally grateful that he shouldered it. From anything as simple as "What do you want to eat" to things as complicated as "What time do you need to be at your psychiatrist appointment," he handled it all.

He took me where I needed to go.

He spoke for me when I could not speak.

Maybe trauma does not fuck with all people's heads like it did with mine. Maybe some people can go through the worst of it and come out the side with a sense of safety and trust. I once told my husband that I never feel safe.

And I still do not.

Thirty plus years later, in some instances I am right back to the moments when I want to end it all. I fight every single day to go into the world and make meaningful contributions. If I had my way, I think I would lock all my doors, close all my curtains and hole up day in and day out.

Every time I do not feel safe, which we have established is always, I spiral back to the helplessness I felt when the Thing happened, and it may as well be happening all over again.

It is exhausting.

I find myself in the depths of despair so often, fading away into it, and to be honest sometimes I just want to let it win. It is just easier. You know, I think about being in a zombie apocalypse far more often than I should—which is to say that I should not think of it at all, but it creeps into my mind on a daily basis. Forget the Roman Empire question: how often are we thinking about an apocalypse?

I know it seems like I just brought up zombies out of nowhere, but I swear it is relevant and I have a point—and that point is that I think about how hard people fight to stay alive in those post-apocalyptic, zombie-infested, skin-being-ripped-from-the-bones scenarios with humans turning on one another in the worst way and I think, "Why are they fighting to stay alive?"

This probably borders a kind of psychosis (do not worry, I will unpack that with my therapist), but I already feel like I am living in a zombie land. At any moment I could be eaten alive by people, I am already struggling to trust. Those I love are just one bite and fever away from turning against me, and it sucks.

The thing about being a partner to someone with a mental illness is that it takes a certain strength. One that often goes unnoticed and underappreciated. I find myself wondering what it is like for my husband to be married to me because, honestly, I do not think I could be married to me.

My depression comes on without warning. I cannot trust people—but, so help me God, I am working on trusting myself.

BYE, FELICIA

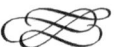

Let us talk podcasts. I am really late to the game on enjoying the concept. I honestly do not know when they began, but I feel like it was definitely in the mid-2010s. They seemed geared mostly towards sci-fi fans and true crime junkies.

When your brain is an unsolved mystery, neither of those options sounds appealing. My journey to podcasts is a long one, so I will attempt to long-story-short here. Let us just say that I was invited to be on a podcast for Love Will Foundation, and I spent an hour talking about a topic I loved and then I realized why podcasts were so appealing. Well, being on them was appealing. I still did not get the draw to listening to other people talk when I am the one who loves to chat.

But then came a pandemic, and what else was there to do but deep dive into podcasts? I spent a year saying that I would listen to podcasts, but I could never find one that sounded appealing. Listening to people talk for an hour. Boring. Anyway, my self-improvement self decided to bail on podcasts and go for the getting-back-to-books route, and I heard a lot about a particular memoir by Glennon Doyle. I hopped on

Amazon and ordered myself a copy of *Untamed,* and when it arrived I read it cover to cover in two days. I could not put it down.

And then I found Glennon on Instagram. And then she said she was launching a podcast, and all my worlds were circling together. I was drawn to her delicious persona and searched for *We Can Do Hard Things* on Spotify. I binged a lot of episodes, and one in particular hit me like a sack of bricks. In an episode, she tells a story: the story of going to see a Van Gogh exhibit. She and her family go to some fancy exhibit, and when they go in they think, *sure, it is fine but definitely over-rated.* They spend their time in the hall and leave only to find out that they never actually entered the exhibit. They were in the entryway. They had to go in deeper into the building to get to the actual exhibit. They saw something good when they could have experienced something grand. They did not know it until after the fact.

I go through phases where I am eternally grateful for my husband seeing that I am more than mental illness and admire him for taking our vows "in sickness and in health" to heart. And then I go through phases where I feel so sorry for him and the fact that he has spent the last twenty years with a person who makes life so hard for him. Who questions his loyalty and the sincerity of his words. I cannot help but think that he has wasted his life on the wrong person. I imagine an alternate reality where he met someone who can bring more to the table. More joy and stability. That is the thing about depression—it manipulates your entire being into believing, no, knowing, that you are the problem.

I want to be hopelessly in love. I want blinded-by-passion type love. In my head, that is. Because offer that to me in reality, and I shut down. I think it is part of the fallout from the Thing. I long for and crave intimacy and vulnerability, but I cannot seem to bring down the walls that will allow me to experience it. Somewhere along the line, my brain equated vulnerability with abuse and intimacy with manipulation. Needless to say, I feel abusive and manipulative or abused and manipulated when those factors are introduced into a situation. It does make me sad. I feel like I am missing out on the best part of marriage, and I am keeping my husband from experiencing it as well. I mean, there must be a certain level of those elements in our marriage because we have five kids, but to say that I have built a house of walls is an understatement.

I worry that I am spending my life, and more specifically marriage, in the Van Gogh exhibit entryway. Sure, it is great, but I sense there should be more. I want to go into the hall with all the pieces, yet I either cannot find my way to the door or I am too scared to walk through it. I am standing in front of my husband, blocking his way into the exhibit. At some moments, I look at him and realize he spent a lot of money on those tickets, and he should be able to get his money's worth. So I tell him I will be ready to walk through the doorway in a minute, but I know it is a lie. Because even though I want to walk through, my feet will not propel me forward. He does not know what he is missing either because he has not seen the full sha-bang. So his "No, Sara, don't do that to yourself" responses are muttered by someone who does not know what he is missing.

When I became suicidal, part of me thought that it was heroic. He was not going to leave me on his own accord. No matter how many times I told him he should. He was going to waste his life and his time in the corridor. He is loyal to a fault. Removing myself from the situation was the only way to give him the chance at more. He should not have to suffer the consequences of my pain.

"You need to leave me." It is always so hard for me to muster these words because I do not want to say them, but at the same time I feel selfish for keeping them in.

"What are you talking about?" This conversation usually catches my husband off guard. It probably also grates on his nerves, but when I bring it up, I mean it. I think of the saying, "If you love someone, let them go," and I think I am being valiant and kind. Releasing him from his obligation of living with a sick person who just makes life hard.

"I make your life harder than it needs to be. I am not your landing space so you can come home and forget about the stresses of the world. I am your stress in the world."

"No, Sara. Don't do that to yourself." I really don't know if he means it, but I know he is a loyal human, so I figure he says it out of a misplaced sense of commitment rather than a place of being hopelessly in love.

That is the thing about depression. It is a liar. It makes you believe that life is miserable because you are in it. There is no mind over matter with depression because it is your mind that is sick. I spend a lot of time wondering if my depression will become fatal. If I will have the continued strength to fight it. If I will even know when it is taking me over. Much like I have learned how to manage the triggers from the Thing that send me spiraling, so have I learned which thoughts are lying to me. Those thoughts are loud and obnoxious, almost deafening, but in the background there are whispers. Quiet inner voices or thoughts, if you will, that all the aforementioned is untrue. That I can work on bringing my walls down. That I will one day make it into the exhibit and it will be glorious. I have learned to focus on those whispers. I used to think they were the liars, but I have come to learn that it is the whispers that speak the truth.

So, when your mind is yelling at you to quit, listen for the quiet voice. The quiet voice is the one worth listening to. I have gotten to a point where I am working on replacing "You need to leave me" with "Thank you for loving me." The quiet voice told me that I could rewire my brain if I wanted to and, God, do I want to.

FEELERS

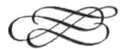

Depression, for me, is not about feeling sad. In fact, I do not feel sad at all. I quite literally feel nothing.

Nada.

Niente.

Oftentimes I test out the black hole. I usually do that through music because I want to feel something. I want to feel romance or joy or sadness or just something.

My Spotify playlist is not for everyone. Actually, people who listen to it—such as my husband—usually mutter the words:

"Your music is so depressing."

But in my head, we have this epic conversation where I respond with a:

"I just like to get into my feelings."

And then because my husband is such a curious mate, he will offer up genuine: "Why?"

Then I will come back with an ever so prophetic: "To make sure I'm still having them."

And then I can see him peering into my soul and understanding my heart better and feeling seen.

But I am still working out that whole vulnerability thing. You know, when you let your spouse see you. Instead, I just smile, look away, and retreat into my head, where all the best conversations take place because I have carved out a safe place in my brain. Where I can let my guard down and be vulnerable and where that vulnerability is cared for. The good news is that I am feeling now, or at least I am trying to.

Despite what it sounds like, I am not crazy. I am just not yet brave enough to feel out loud.

But maybe one day I will be.

FINDING FAITH

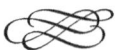

The competition for my soul has been a lifelong battle. I
spent many years insisting that I believed in God, and
that was enough. I did not want to claim that I was either
Christian or Muslim; I was faithful. I have a relationship with
God, after all, I believe in him. As time went on, I felt there was
a void, one that no one could fill.

There was an overwhelming fear associated with accepting
Jesus Christ as my Savior. I disregarded it at every
turn. Throughout my life, I had several friends who attempted
to convert me to Christianity. I saw them as cult members. I
pitied them for being sucked into the lie. However, they
planted a seed.

I was married in a Catholic church. I refused to say:

"In the name of the Father, the Son and the Holy Spirit."

I did not believe in the Holy Trinity, and I did not want to
say something born of tradition. To this day, I regret that
choice.

I knew going into my marriage that we would raise our
children Catholic. I wanted them to have a solid faith, as I felt

that was always missing from my foundation. When our first son was born, my husband wanted him baptized. As the baptism got closer, my feet got colder. I went through with it, but I felt like a deceiver.

I did not feel as opposed to our daughter's baptism; I saw it as a nice celebration, but I refused to put a bonnet on her. To me, I was taking the stance that I did not fully embrace this idea and would not conform to these rituals.

However, after her baptism, something changed. God went to work full time on my heart. I kept being brought back to the notion that I needed to accept Jesus Christ. I mulled over this for six months before I acknowledged God was truly calling to me as he had for the last twenty years.

The bellow was too loud. I telephoned my sister.

"I feel like I need to accept Jesus."

Silence on the other end. And then tears.

"Sara, last night I prayed in our prayer group that my family would open their hearts to Jesus."

Goosebumps. The timing seemed incredible.

"I don't know what I am supposed to do next."

"I can say a prayer with you to accept Jesus."

"Oh, no, I can't do that. I do not know that I really believe it. I feel like a liar."

"You just need to say it."

I could not. This was not the time. I spent the next several months trying to open my heart and to gather the words. Every time I came close to saying it, a deafening voice would consume my thoughts. I thought God was speaking to me. It would shout:

"You are a liar."

"I'm not a liar. I think I really believe this."

A quiet reassurance.

"Yes, you do."

An aggressive contradiction:

"No, you are just a liar."

Maybe I am. I could not say the words, but I could not stop thinking about them either. I want to say them.

Overwhelming fear consumed me. Another loud, insistent thought:

"If you do this, something bad will happen to your children."

What if God tests me after I accept Jesus to prove my faith? What if he takes my children from me to teach me a lesson? I love my children too much to risk their lives for my soul.

A quiet encouragement:

"Nothing will happen."

I did not believe the meager attempts of my thoughts to comfort me.

The shouting returned.

"Not only will something bad happen to your children, but it will be at your hand."

I was evil. I knew I was. I was a liar trying to say I believed in a God I did not. I was someone who was capable of hurting those I loved the most. I spent the next several months hating myself; feeling unworthy of a love that was being offered freely. I could not stop my thoughts from consuming me.

I looked at my kids...

... Over and over.

No, I would never hurt them. I am not capable of it. I want to accept Jesus.

The closer I came to saying the words, the more I yearned to ignore the hateful and discouraging feelings. They were promoting fear and doubt. The quiet voice never wavered.

I accepted Jesus.

The roaring, angry thoughts immediately and forever fell silent.

That was the moment I realized that the enemy is loud and forceful. He disguises his voice as truth, manipulating us into believing the worst to be true.

The voice of the Holy Spirit is the one that speaks to us in the calm. That soothes us in the quiet.

It is imperative that we discern between the two.

TEMP TAGS

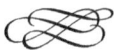

I want to be my kids' safe space, I want to calm their storms, but I think sometimes I partake in their chaos.

I know I am the adult and supposed to be mature, but I also have anxiety and sometimes that is a savage animal that takes over my rational brain, and I am reacting before I can get my bearings to think.

This one time, I was sitting with my husband in my spot and my baby girl came and squeezed herself in between us. We were both wearing hoodies; she grabbed our hoodie strings and tied them together. "There, now you are soulmates forever."

"Do you think we are soulmates?" I asked her.

"You are the best soulmates," she responded.

It has gotten me thinking about the concept of soulmates. I have always thought the idea was bogus. A soulmate suggests a divine intervention, a greater plan put into place long before I walked into the room where I saw my husband sitting in a corner chair strumming on a guitar for the first time. When he looked up from his guitar and directly at me, for a moment, it felt like the rest of the world melted away and all he saw was me. That aura of confidence faded pretty quickly, and the insecurities crept in not too long after.

Sometimes I wish I savored that moment more. I think back on it now and wonder what he thought. I have always been too afraid to ask. I prefer the version of the story where romance trumps just mere curiosity about who has entered a room. Where it's more than just the coincidence of two people running into each other and making a series of choices leading to a commitment that surpasses magic. I have almost found the concept offensive, as if I did not have any control over what happens next in my relationship. It all happens by chance.

Moreover, I really do not like reminders that life is fleeting or temporary. That our time one day will end. We all know it, but when we are reminded by actually losing someone it just seems like an unnecessary reminder. It does not so much bother me that my life will end as much as it does that the life of those around me will. It makes me feel scared and insecure. It makes me want to hunker down and never leave the house. Worse yet, never let my husband and kids leave. It is so terrifying to even contemplate that this life we created could be shattered within seconds that my brain shuts down at the mere thought of it.

And that is why I usually curl under my husband's armpit anytime he is sitting on the couch or lounging in bed. It is my love language. It makes me feel safe and shielded from the chaos in my mind. But we did this thing where we had kids, a whole crew of them; five, to be exact. And it turns out that they also want to curl under his armpit in my spot and snuggle.

Rude.

I suppose he holds the key to calm. I know for a fact that I do not. For example, my son recently asked my husband:

"Are you ever worried that your beard will grow into your mouth and you'll swallow it?"

"No."

"Why not?"

"Because I am not afraid of that."

What do you mean, you are not afraid of the improbable? My psyche has been built on the basis that the improbable and the unlikely are just a hop, skip, and jump away from infiltrating my reality.

Sometimes I wonder what it is like to be free of irrational thoughts. To just be able to live in the here and now without your mind wandering to all the horrific things that could occur, and then your mind running with it, and before you know it, the tears are flowing because you have spiraled an unlikely-to-happen scenario into probability—and every ounce of security that you spent the last twenty years fighting for has left you.

Here is what I am learning: when your brain starts up with the intrusive thoughts and you recognize it, get up and go outside. Take a deep breath. Feel fresh air in your lungs and remember that, in this moment, you are safe and everything is okay.

Life may be fast, fleeting, and temporary, but so are panic attacks.

SUIT UP

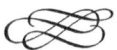

I recently confessed to my husband that I have been a mess, and I think I have been a mess because of all the walls that I spent a lifetime building—well, I am finally curious enough to see what happens when I tear them down.

This is my "burn it all down" phase, I guess, but spoiler alert: I am busting at the seams with insecurity.

It is weird. I feel more myself and more alive than I ever have. I am confident and strong, and let me tell you *that* is not the person who has been walking earthside for the last three decades. A rebirth of sorts has taken place, and in being born again I am entering the world sans armor and, God, I hope they like me.

It was easier when I armored up after the Thing. If people did not like the way I spoke, I changed it. When they made fun of my laugh for sounding too high-pitched, I cultivated it into a deeper-toned, more-pleasing-to-the-senses chuckle. If they did not like my style, I went shopping. If they did not like my jokes, I adjusted the punch line. As a result, people liked me, but I did not like myself.

Now I am walking around with my heart on my sleeve, being told that I should be cautious with that because not everyone is good and, man, do I know that already—and I have decided to wear my heart on my sleeve anyway.

I was explaining this to my husband and I got to the crux of the matter when I confessed: "I'm afraid I have changed too much and you won't like me anymore." He said the thing that you want your lover to say, which is: *"Sara, I have always seen who you were when you weren't trying, and I love you."*

Obviously, he must have his own issues loving someone as broken as me, but I would be lying if I did not say that I have since replayed that moment and his words in my head hundreds of times, utilizing his words as my new-found armor.

PEOPLE PERSON

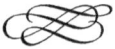

Sometimes your person will not support all your dreams.
Sometimes your person will not be there with open
arms when you so desperately need to be held.

Sometimes your person will leave when you have asked
them to stay.

Sometimes your person will not get it.

Sometimes your person will say what you do not want to
hear—what you do not need to hear.

That does not make them not your person.

Sometimes our people need grace to be human too.

DECISIONS, DECISIONS

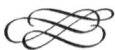

I recently saw where a big-time influencer announced she was getting divorced. She referenced an article she'd written about how she and her husband could get through anything, and how obviously that was no longer true—but how she'd believed it when she wrote it. Gosh, I love her for that perspective, but I think that's why I do not write about my marriage often. I do not feel comfortable sharing how I am going to choose my husband every day for the rest of my life. I guess standing in front of our closest friends and family members echoing our vows is not what I call commitment. Writing about it on the internet is, and that kind of commitment scares the daylights out of me.

When I became engaged to Lance, my dad said, *"You're too young. What if you grow apart?"* and I responded with the most naïve, *"But what if we grow together?"* As innocent as that response was, I have used it as the road map in my marriage, but that has not kept me immune from doubt.

We have almost thrown in the towel quite a few times, and in those moments I felt relief. I could finally stop worrying about when he was going to leave and wondering what straw would break the camel's metaphorical back. The moment had finally arrived, and I could wallow in the outcome that had always been my destiny. Who knows, maybe that is still how our story will end.

Or maybe I will choose him for another day, and he will choose me for one more. This marriage thing only works when we choose each other even when we do not want to, day after day, choice after choice. Even when it is hard and messy. Especially then.

Maybe we cannot say for sure what the outcome of our relationships will be. All we can do is be honest with ourselves and each other as to what we believe to be true in the present moment.

Sometimes love is organically romantic and sometimes you will lose yourself in your lover's eyes, yet in reality love is a choice, one that can be tedious at times. I know that sounds cliché, but I think what ends more relationships is looking for magic instead of making it.

THE OTHER F-WORD

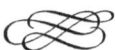

My body has changed over the years. It has taken me a lot of time, repetition, and reassurance to love the skin I inhabit. I guess it is the fact that skinny is in. I mean, not too skinny, obviously, because that is gross. There is a right kind of skinny. When things do not bulge where they should not and you do not have stretchmarks in places that no one knew could stretch.

I was that kind of skinny before. At the detriment of my mental health and, to be honest, probably my overall health. I was never skinny enough to be considered clinically anorexic, but I stopped eating. And I did not make myself throw up on the rare occasion that I did eat, so I was not considered bulimic; I just drank as much diet coke and sweet n low-flavored drinks as I could because they had this magical diuretic effect, and it made my stomach go from bulky to flat in no time at all. I did not spend all my time in a gym setting, but I would lock myself in my room with a stack of hardcover books on top of my stomach and proceed to do—literally—one thousand crunches per day. When I caved into hunger and exhaustion, I hated myself. And when I was strong enough to avoid food and put my body through the ringer, well, I hated myself.

It got to the point where my body rejected food. At least that is how it felt. Any time I ate, I would become violently ill with sharp stomach cramps and bodily fluids being excreted from the upper and lower GI tracts. The only time I did not get sick while eating was when I got pregnant. I remember thinking that was weird. Maybe my body just knew that it had to take the nutrients or someone else would suffer. I am a lot of things, but I am not "the bad guy." I maintained a pretty svelte figure for about three years post baby number 5. And then I heard about intuitive eating.

I will be honest: I cannot claim that I am an intuitive eater in the research sense, but based on what I know about the word intuitive, I am an intuitive eater. It all happened around the end of 2019. I started putting on weight; I probably put on 40 pounds before the COVID- 20 was ever a thing, and then COVID added another 30, so essentially I am up 70 pounds from the weight I was at twenty-two. To be honest, I do not feel like I am living in a larger body. I actually feel kind of good. I eat food I enjoy and food I crave. I do not eat when my stomach gives my brain a full cue—unless Aunty Flo is on the verge of a visit, then, forget it, bring on the chocolate and all bets are off.

Lately, and by lately I mean since free shipping with Amazon Prime became a fad, I have been online shopping. Especially for clothing. Especially since everyone and their brother has been popping up with boutiques. I rarely ever enter a store anymore to try on clothing, but over the last two years I have upgraded my closet sizes from medium to large tops and from size 8 to size 12 pants. I even think my feet got bigger. It seems like my shoe size went up by at least a size, so there is that. Anyway, I usually shop sales, and I usually do so when I am feeling the need for a closet refresh. My most recent package arrived, and I eagerly tried things on. The first piece was a sea-foam-green, deep-V-neck, dolman-sleeved, just-the-right-amount-above-the-knee dress. And it fit like a chef's kiss glove.

But for some reason, I saw myself in the mirror for the first time. Like really saw myself. I mean, I have noticed hanging flesh and loose tummy skin. Afterall, I have had five kids, I knew I was all-around bigger, but when I looked down I could still see my feet, so I did not really notice how much weight I'd piled on. But that dress, cute as it was, gave me this kind of reality check. Like my stomach is big. So is my backside. All around and in general, I am big. More than big; I am, gulp, fat.

That is an f-word that has always made me cringe. Whether someone was using it to describe themselves or another, it gave me a shhhhh-we-do-not-say-that vibe. I would be lying if I said the idea of stringent exercise and restrictive meal planning has not crossed my mind since the weight crossed my hips. I wonder if my husband still finds me attractive because even when he says he does, I roll my eyes since obviously he is lying. I cannot help but think that it is actually not about him, it is about me. And where I place my values.

When I do my yoga and drink water when I am thirsty, and eat what my body is asking for, I feel so good. When I ignore my body's requests for movement and nutrition, I feel lousy. We have an instinct to tell people they are not fat if they say they are. Why is it such a dirty word? Who says that less curves are more desirable? I am fat, and I rocked that green dress. There is no shame in allowing my body to change because I have changed. I am not the same frail, insecure, self-loathing twenty-three-year-old girl I was. I actually can go for hours without feeling afraid and lost. Sometimes I even feel like I have myself together. If growing up means growing wide, then I am here for it.

This body that allows me to experience this life is an awesome temple, and it really does not matter if that makes the world uncomfortable. Maybe our bodies get bigger as we get older because we learn how to take up more space. So, yeah, I am fat. And I am going to fight the urge to qualify or justify the use of that word. I am fat, and I add value to the spaces I am in. I may not always think it—but, I will *always* believe it.

Maybe to some (including myself from time to time) I look like I have let myself go by putting on some weight.

And I guess I have let myself go.

But in truth, I am lighter.

I have let go of the weight of overwhelming shame, constant fear, and all-consuming doubt.

It is not the same body it was 70 pounds ago, and neither am I.

So, if you are like me and cringe at your reflection, look again.

And again.

Until you see it.

That your body is beautiful exactly as it is because it tells the story of all your yesterdays and that, warrior, is a story worth telling.

UNTOLD CHILDREN'S STORIES

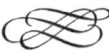

I no longer talk about my kids when I write online. I used to when their problems were small and simpler, like finding the balance between their need for snuggle time and my need for down time, or how to juggle their nap time with my needing-to-vacuum time.

As the years have gone on, it has gotten harder to tell our stories. Mostly because I teeter on the line between telling my story as a parent and telling their story as humans.

As they get older, the challenges get bigger. While I would love to share for the sake of those struggling to navigate these treacherous waters, I find myself falling silent.

Believe it or not, I do have some boundaries when it comes to what I will write about on the worldwide web, and I thought I would take this opportunity to explain myself.

In fact, there are two things I do not share intimate details on my Rebel Housewife adventures, and those two things are:

My kids and my marriage. I mean, other than what is in this book of course.

Let me go ahead and just give a disclaimer to the effect that this is just my opinion and I am not judging anyone who has different boundaries than mine.

For someone who shares such deep, dark, personal information, you would think that my parenting journey—more realistically, struggles—and my marriage ups and downs—because all marriages have ups and downs—would be fair fodder.

Let me tell you a quick back story that will circle back to my point.

I *think*.

Last night I had the best time with my #1. We made dinner and talked.

That is it, and I loved every moment of it. I looked at his eyes and his expressions and listened to his changing voice and thought:

"*This is the good stuff.*"

But during our conversation, he told me about a YouTube video he watched in which the creators were doing some sort of spicy-chicken-wing challenge. One of them ate a wing so spicy it made his mouth bleed.

I said, "*Did you say bleed?!!*"

Guys. I am not lying. He confirmed that he did indeed say *bleed*.

I looked at him with sincere shock and said, "*Why on earth would anyone do that?*"

You know what he said with an ever-so-casual shrug? He said: "*Content.*"

And there you have it.

After I made him swear up and down that he would never do anything for the sake of "content" or views or popularity and gave a pretty lengthy speech on where we can find fulfillment—and, spoiler alert, it is not on mindless YouTube videos—I decided this is everything that is wrong in this world.

In a nutshell, this is why I will not write about my kids.

They are not content.

But I am a wordy writer, so I am going to exit the nutshell and elaborate.

I think this is something all creators struggle with. Finding the line between privacy and authenticity. I think that privacy might be a combination of respect and fear.

Now you are probably thinking that I must not respect myself because I do not keep many personal trials and tribulations private. But if we are going to play that game, then I guess I would say that actually I am fearless when it comes to sharing my story.

When it comes to my kids, it is different. Because it is not just my story. It is not just about me. It is me intersected with them.

Maybe they do not want to share their stories and, also, they are not old enough to know what the consequences of sharing online are, so I do not ask them for their permission to alleviate my conscience.

Instead, I just take it off the table.

I usually ask myself if the story I am about to tell is something I would have wanted my mom to share about me with strangers when I was that age, and usually the answer is no.

My kids should not be expected to have a different emotional response to sharing their struggles, which is basically what I equate to sharing my parenting struggles.

It is how I am helping them navigate *their* deep waters.

See? Intertwined.

And then the fear aspect.

If I say something completely generic, like:

"All parents struggle."

I feel like I would hear a resounding YES from the rooftops.

If I gave a specific example of *how* I struggle as a parent, I feel like I would hear a slew of unsolicited advice along with opinions and feedback that would clutter my already loud thoughts.

When I told the stories of breast versus bottle, or cry it out versus co-sleeping, it was easy to read through everyone's thoughts and even manage the criticism because, in the end, we overall agreed that fed was best, and that as long as our babies were sleeping everything was okay.

Their most basic needs were being met, and at the end of the day we were all getting them where they needed to be.

But kids do not stay basic for long.

In fact, they turn into complex human beings with complicated questions that become harder to answer.

With needs that become harder to meet.

It stops being about meeting needs and becomes about also meeting values.

And we all have different values. I think if we all looked at the core of our value system, we would realize they are actually very similar.

We want our kids to be safe.

We want our kids to be happy.

We want our kids to be loved.

We want our kids to be free.

I think our goals are the same, and that we just find so many different ways to say the same thing that we begin to think we are all singing a different melody when in fact we are in harmony.

I do not talk about my kids much anymore or our struggles

or our conversations; they are so deeply personal and so deeply tied to who we are at our core that it does not matter what anyone else would do.

It matters what we would do.

And, unpopular opinion, but sometimes we do not need the world to validate our decisions or praise us for them. Sometimes we just need our kids to know sincerely and deeply we love and adore them. Sometimes I think that sharing them online takes that security away from them.

And that is a line I am not willing to cross.

So, I will keep it generic.

You will not find me giving the *how* I am struggling *but* I am willing to stand up and say:

Parenting is hard. And exhausting. And it is a struggle. And we *all* are struggling. And if we are not yet, we will soon. And we will handle each situation the best we know how. And if we did not do what could be our best this time, we will try to be better next time.

Because we are parents.

And that is what we do.

REJECTIMONY

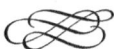

I t's hard, you know. When you see people getting the things you want. It makes you ask a lot of hard questions, like, *"Why can't it be me?" "Why can't I have that?"*

The jealousy can really eat a person up from the inside out. It is worse when we try to pretend that we aren't filled with envy. The more I try to act happy for someone when I am really seething with envy, the harder it is for me to really be happy for them. And we have associated jealousy with being a bad person, so we don't want to admit we feel it and the cycle perpetuates itself. But here's the thing: we are not our feelings.

I have two kids who play soccer competitively, and by competitively I mean they compete with each other. They are good. I mean really good.

My #4 is a natural talent. She one day woke up and decided she wanted to be on a soccer team, scored six goals in her first game and has gone on to just get better and better. Don't get me wrong, she works her tail off, but she has this halo around her that just makes things come easy to her.

My #3 is me. He is also a natural talent who works his butt off. But the opportunities that have presented themselves to my #4 have not appeared to him... yet.

Every time he learns that his sister is being recognized, he takes it as a personal attack. Like there's only so many good soccer players and her level of good diminishes his level since they can't both be good.

And I have tried to tell him how untrue that philosophy is. I have told him it is not a competition. You don't need to feel jealous. Her awards don't take away from your skills. And so on and so on.

Then it dawned on me. I have only been upping the ante on his envy. Jealousy is gaining momentum with each "don't" I sputter toward him. I finally decided to be honest with him.

"*Look,*" I said. "*I know it's hard, and I know what it feels like to be jealous.*"

I picked up a book that I recently began reading. "*You see this book? I didn't want to read it. I sent them my story and they wouldn't include it in the book, and look how many authors made it in here. Man, that was hard for me. But you know what? Since then I have gotten my own book deal. Someone is publishing my words. So celebrate her time because you will have yours.*"

Literally a smile came to his lips, and he in the lightest of tones said, "*Okay.*"

And I felt his relief.

All I am trying to say is: acknowledge what you feel, and acknowledge it without judgment. Because I guarantee someone else out there is feeling it. When you bring those feelings to the light, they just lose all their heavy. It brings all the relief. And you can get on with it.

I bought the book.

I read the book.

I loved the book.

And I knew that was not where my story was meant to be told... yet.

TUNNEL VISION

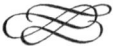

L ife is weird.

On my couch, with my head back on the cushions and hands over my eyes, I was trying to block out the chitter-chatter happening around me and mulling over some topics I wanted to write about on my blog over the coming week. I set up my Mental Health Mondays, Tuesday Re-Runs and Thursday Thoughts as a way to guide what I write about. Essentially to make my life easier and narrow the billions of ideas in my head down to thousands of ideas.

I am never quite sure how real to be when tackling mental-health-related topics. I think I have made it clear throughout these pages that sharing the actual nitty-gritty of living with depression and anxiety might be too much and potentially triggering to others. Balancing authenticity with mindfulness is tricky.

Then I thought about one of the healing practices I have found—like tattoo therapy—and realized I did not want to talk about healing. Being on a healing journey means that sometimes you are experiencing the peaks of healing and sometimes you are in the valleys of it. At this particular time, I was in the valley. I closed my laptop and resumed my position with head against the back of the couch, eyes closed, while wishing I had my phone and headphones so I could turn on my Spotify writing playlist, but my youngest child had hijacked said phone and I either get quiet time to write while she plays games or not. There is no simultaneous quiet time for her and Spotify for me.

In some ways, I am fearless in sharing my story, but really, when I think about it, I am fearless in sharing what I have overcome. I am not fearless in sharing what I am currently going through. Usually because I do not have any answers. I do not know how it is going to end, and I do not know what I am going to do. I know that it *will* end, and I *will* get better, but the details are fuzzy until I have been able to process it all.

As I was sitting with my head back, my youngest son asked, "*What are you doing?*"

To be honest, I was annoyed with his question and I replied with an aggravated and slightly whiny, "*I'm thinking about what to write.*" He followed up my response and said, "*Can I help you think of something?*"

I reluctantly (*and probably*) unkindly said, "*Sure*" when what I really wanted to say was "*Go away.*" And he said, "*You could write about tattoos.*" And that made me pause, pop my head up and look in his big blue eyes with impossibly long blond lashes and *notice* him.

And his precious heart.

I responded to his perfect timing with, "*I was actually considering writing about that.*"

And if this were a scripted moment on a television show like *This is Us,* he would have said something like, "*Well, you should then*" and he would have sweetly galloped away, and I would have the most prophetic words pouring out of me.

But this is not television.

Instead, I am telling you *this* story. The one about how you can be seen by your people even when you feel invisible if you just take the time to notice.

What was I going through?

Nothing major. I was just experiencing living with depression and anxiety. I think my depression is overall well controlled, but I do find myself in the ebb and flow of feeling hopeless and numb. Moments where I do not take the time to really sit down and process what that means for me.

Why? No reason. I just don't.

Wellness is hard. It takes effort. And usually it takes the most effort when you do not have any to offer. Even though wellness feels harder, it also feels better.

Wellness feels better.

When I am in the middle of feeling my feelings or lack thereof, I usually feel alone and like no one gets me or my depression with insurmountable anxiety, and I get tired of talking about it. I think to myself that they have heard it all before, and they do not want to keep hearing it. It must be disheartening to always hear how your person is on some mental-health tightrope and you are never quite sure how well they can balance the act.

Instead, I say nothing and (*kind of*) suffer in silence, but misery loves company.

I think that when we are silent, we open the door to let our minds ravage our thoughts and tell us lies. I think we are angry at those around us for not seeing that we are struggling. But on the flip side, when they ask how we are doing, we say, "*Fine*" and, really, we do not want to talk about it. We want to be left alone.

But sometimes—just sometimes—someone will intercept our thoughts and ask if they can join us where we are. Sometimes we will let them. We will not shout, "*Go away*" but instead we will reluctantly say, 'Sure," and then they will say something in such a way that we *know* we are seen, loved and cared for. And while they may not know the depth of our struggle, they know what helps us regain our footing, and they offer it as a gentle reminder. In those moments, we can decide if we will take that offering and tuck it away in the back of our minds, and continue to be ravaged by our illness—or recognize it as a powerful invitation to let the walls down, share that which haunts us and continue on our path of healing.

In the words of Glennon Doyle: we can do hard things.

And to add my own little flair to G's words: but we cannot do them alone. So let your people in. Even when you do not want to. Let their offerings be the light at the end of the long, dark, seemingly endless tunnel because if there is one thing I have learned in this journey with depression it is this: the tunnel *will* end and that there is always, always, *always* a light at the end of it.

TIPPY TONES

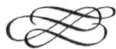

Winter can be hard. There are snow days, and sick days, and gray days, and the whole "being a parent" thing and having to meet your kids' needs.

Days of endless wintry mixes that shut down all the nearby towns and keep kids home—indoors for days on end leave little time for self. Many times that sends me into a tizzy because while my kids are best friends—they can also fight like boxing champions when we are trapped indoors and unable to play outside in ice like they can in snow.

Although, some winter days are not like that. They are actually pretty chill. I mean, everyone still loses their bearings by 4:00 p.m., the witching hour, when dinner needs to be made and all hell breaks loose. But the days, overall, can be nice. It was the kind of day where you want to post on social media lots of pictures of mani-pedis, arts and crafts, baking, and snuggles.

It makes me think: why are some snow days miserable while others are magical?

And I think that I am the reason.

When my girls ask me to paint their nails first thing in the morning, before I even had coffee, I would usually say:

"No. I want to drink my coffee, and then I'll paint your nails."

Then they proceed to ask me one hundred million times, *"Are you done yet,"* and I get so annoyed that I cannot drink my coffee in peace and quiet. By the time I get to their nails, we are all combative and crabby.

Sometimes, I say *"Sure"* before coffee and then this weird thing happens: they leave me alone, and I drink my coffee in peace and quiet. On this particular day I thought to myself, *"Why do I not always respond this way?"* I began to look around and think even more. My current environment consisted of counters covered in construction paper and markers, my little ones had set up a little craft corner in the living room, there were dried up Play-Doh scraps all over the kitchen floor and game boxes lined up along the hallway walls.

That usually sends me into another tizzy. Mess and clutter are ginormous anxiety provoking triggers.

But that day I thought, *"Who cares? We live here."*

I have said that before, and I have tried to accept it and honor it, but my mind is usually always like: *"Clean up, clean up, clean up."*

That day, I did not. I baked instead. And I focused on dishes and the laundry because clean sinks and empty hampers help me manage my clutter claustrophobia. And it was fine.

I was calm, they were calm.

And then that got me thinking even more. How much I set the tone in my house. And I hate to admit that on the days when I am irritable and anxious, my kids seem to fight and nag more. They pick up what I put down.

And then that got me thinking even more, more. How important it is that I lay down whatever I am going through to be there for them. I cannot be a physically present and emotionally available mom when I am already filled to the brim with my own battles.

And that made the figurative light bulb in my head illuminate: that's why self-care matters.

Yoga and journaling and devotionals and meditation and blogging. These are the things that keep me sane. They sort out my thoughts. They free up my internal clutter. And when I have more inside space, I can allow for more things to come in.

Like my people's needs.

And my kids telling me jokes and playing games with them. I have more capacity for spider monkey snuggles and for following endless sticky note treasure hunts. I am able to walk them through big emotions that are usually what leads to all the fighting because let us be real, if I can barely handle my big emotions, of course they struggle to handle theirs.

So a thought for us anxious parents: we have to do the things that calm us so we can have the space to calm them.

After all, it is a disservice to our people if we do not manage our internal chaos. They need us to give them outer peace so they can foster their inner peace.

It is not about giving up on yourself or losing yourself. And it is definitely not about sacrificing things that make you you. It is about making space. It is about putting your needs aside momentarily so you can meet theirs. And then remembering that to do it all again tomorrow, you have to go to the side and pick your needs back up—and because you have been there all day for them, they will gladly sit on the sidelines while you are there for you.

Your people want you to be okay. And at the end of the

day, don't we just all want some peace... and definitely some quiet?

ROOTING FOR WINGS

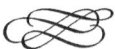

Y ou know what I have been thinking about?

This meme or post or quote I once saw on Facebook that said in huge bold letters something to the effect of:

"DON'T YELL AT YOUR KIDS AND THEN EXPECT THEM TO HAVE A GOOD DAY."

And when I saw it, my initial reaction was, *"That's a really good point."*

And it impacted me in such a way that I felt guilty each time there was conflict with my children in the mornings. However, while getting five kids ready for school every single flipping morning, there is bound to be some kind of conflict.

They either want to sleep in or are mad you did not wake them up earlier. They want to dress for summer in frigid temperatures and vice versa. Brushing their teeth and wearing winter coats are not cool options and asking if they are ready to go can either send them over their metaphorical ledges or be cause for them to gleefully skip to the car to face the day.

And on the days that started essentially as hell in a hand

basket, that saying would pop into my head and I would try to find a way to turn the flailing morning around.

But sometimes—like yesterday—I cannot.

Because a couple of my dear loves had behaviors that demanded consequences. They were disrespectful and rude and belligerent, and you know what? That is just not acceptable.

Why do I feel the eyes of judgment penetrating through the pages as I type this? For some reason, I have it in my head that we are supposed to let our kids feel their feelings and not correct them for it.

Go ahead and cancel me now, because I think that is messed up and I disagree with the sentiment.

Now, here is the thing I tell my kids all the time...

They can *be* angry.

They can *feel* angry.

They can disagree with the rules and not like them.

They can speak up and we can discuss it.

But being angry does not give them the right to be mean.

Or disrespectful or rude or belligerent.

Anyway. I could not get the fruit of my loins to take time and space to feel their feelings and come back to a calmer conversation.

They are young and spry and ready to fight at a moment's notice. Ah, remember having the energy and desire to assert your opinion and win an argument?

I am too old and definitely too tired for that.

Therefore, voices inevitably escalated, and after school grounding-consequences ensued.

I thought, "*They're going to have a bad day today and maybe I shouldn't have told them about their consequences before school and now the tone for their day is going to be a downer and*

I did the one thing some random Facebook post told me not to do:
I sent them to school angry." And, to be honest, I was pretty
upset with myself.

But then I thought, *"Forget that and forget the random*
meme."

Because you know what I believe to be true? Kids need
consequences, and they need boundaries.

Don't they?

We cannot *make* our kids have good days every day.

Can we?

And even if we could... should we?

I don't think so. I kind of think that mentality erases the
human experience. Conflict *will* arise in their lives, and their
actions *will* have consequences.

Why wouldn't we practice that at home? Why wouldn't we
teach them to accept responsibility? Why not teach them how
to navigate the hard things?

Just because we do not want them to feel bad?

I am going to digress for a smidge, but it is going to circle
back—so hang with me.

There is also this saying in marriage: *Don't go to bed angry.*
And again I say, forget that.

Go to bed angry.

And I say that as someone who used to hold on to that
saying like it was the actual Gospel.

I would badger my husband into a resolution of our
conflict, all in the name of not going to bed angry—and you
know what usually happened? We all got angrier.

Sometimes you need time and quiet and to get some
sleep to process the day's events and formulate clear
thoughts.

I mean, we are so focused on instant gratification (*I am*

looking at you, same-day Amazon Prime deliveries) that we have forgotten that it is *all* a process.

Conflict resolution is a process.

And I think we need to give ourselves permission again to take the time to resolve it.

Slow down.

Take a moment or fifty to be angry.

Feel it.

Understand it.

It has taken me nearly four decades to realize that is called self-awareness.

And self-awareness is magical. And healing.

Then when you have that awareness for yourself, you can effectively communicate that to your partner.

And here is where we circle back.

When your kids act out, it is okay to make them slow down and recognize their feelings and not act out in them.

They can have bad days if they have made bad decisions.

It is okay to put them back in line. It is okay to tell them that their behavior is not okay.

So sometimes they are going to go to school mad. Sometimes their mornings are going to be less than desirable and maybe that will set the tone for their day.

Or maybe we teach them that nothing is so catastrophic that they cannot recover. That while they have to accept responsibility for their actions, they are also responsible for their feelings.

They can *choose* to turn a lousy morning around.

They can be held accountable and still be productive.

And they are always loved.

It is not up to us as parents to erase those moments or over-look them because we want them to *feel* good.

I kind of think if we keep in that mindset, then we are going to raise a generation of people who only know how to throw temper tantrums and do not know how to compromise.

They will not know what it means to slow down, and they definitely will be clueless when it comes to working towards real change.

We are going to raise a generation of kids who do not know that what they want is not all that matters. The world does not revolve around our precious people.

I know. Cancel me again.

We are going to raise kids who lack empathy and courage and kindness.

I just think we should love our kids enough to let them have bad days.

Teach them to stop and think.

Show them how to slow down.

But here is the kicker: we, the parents, have to do the same.

So maybe it comes back to the age-old adage: if we want to change the world (*or raise good kids*) then we need to start with ourselves.

BORED GAMES

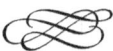

I have been thinking lately that I want to get a living room sign that says, *BE BORED* in big bold italic letters. I want it front and center on an overly plain wall we have at home.

I mentioned this to my daughter, and she said to me in her mocking teenage voice, *"Oh, wow, that's so clever, Mother."* She is not a fan of boredom. I think she comes by it honestly. I have a hard time slowing down. Like, just sitting and not doing anything. Allowing my shoulders to fall and my chest to loosen. My mind to wander and my muscles to relax. I am either on the go or fast asleep. It is hard for me to find the middle ground where I let my mind shut off and soak in the present. I start veering to my to-do list, and then I start getting anxious and have to cross things off the list. I feel like I should always be doing something. I have been trying to let myself be bored. The more I slow down and allow my brain to reset, the less overwhelmed I feel. Even with a lingering laundry list of items that need to be completed, such as laundry.

I do not understand how you can breathe in and out of a

bottle and not have enough air, my son says as he crinkles a water bottle down to nothing by inhaling all the air out of it and then exhaling to blow it back up like a balloon. What wonders can come from curiosity. Let them be bored and let yourself be bored too. Let your mind wander into a blank canvas and see what it can paint.

This book, for example. I have been stumped for weeks as to what more I can possibly say. How I can turn a thought into a story. I am in my car, seat leaned back to the point that I can feel my muscles in my stomach pulling. Listening to a song I cannot get enough of on repeat. One that elicits all the feels. It is pitch-black outside, and my mind is soaking in the stillness of the night. I did not know what to write until I stopped doing things. Until I put the phone down, stopped scrolling and I let myself be still. That is when my mind could wonder and wander. The best ideas are born out of boredom.

Maybe it is time to combat the constant pull we feel towards our newsfeeds. Maybe it is time to put down our devices and take back our boredom. Maybe we stop filling our minds with information on every story at every moment and give our brains time to process what is immediately occurring within our own community. Or maybe start even smaller: what is happening within our own families? Nope; even smaller. What is happening within ourselves? What glorious truths will we discover about our own beautiful souls when we gift ourselves with boredom? And what ripples of beauty will these discoveries send off into the world?

I have been obsessed with this idea of ripples. How we can have an impact that far exceeds our own reach. To be honest, I never thought that was possible—creating a ripple as a human, I mean. I can guarantee that life is not happening within our screens; it is happening behind them and, not to put on pressure or guilt, we are missing it. Boredom births music and poetry and art and lyrics and all the things that make our spirits come to life. What more could a person with mental illness ask for than for their spirit to come to life?

KEEP GOING

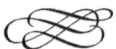

It is Thursday morning. The sky is a crystal-clear blue, the morning is cool and crisp. All in all, my favorite time of the year. I am sitting on my couch between two sicklings, aka my baby boy and baby girl. My blond-haired, blue-eyed, my-genes-are-obsolete child is pacing around the couch and letting me know he is sick by constantly stating, "I don't feel good. I don't feel good."

He finally falls asleep and the silence is golden. My brown-eyed, brown-haired, maybe-my-genes-peeked-through-here three-year-old is as white as the missing clouds. Only lifting her head to weakly proclaim that her tummy hurts. I promptly grab the designated bucket just in the nick of time.

All the while I cannot concentrate on what matters: taking care of my kids. My mind is racing, heart pounding, chest tightening, doom setting in. I have to work today, and I do not know how I am going to make it in. We are lucky we have family nearby to help us in these situations. Yet I cannot help but feel that having two sick kids, one actively spewing out her stomach contents, seems like an unfair time to reach out for help. I do not even like the aftermath clean up in these situations, and I birthed these beauties. They are not quiet, sleeping, sick kids today. They are pacing, crying, puking, demanding a lot of work and emotional energy. Emotional energy that I do not have.

What I know is that the stress, whether real or imagined, of having to call into work or having to ask for help is unbearable. I cannot take a deep breath in; I am floundering in the overwhelming feelings of not being able to care for my kids when I need to and not being a reliable employee to my employer. I am sipping on my thrice-reheated half-caff coffee and searching the internet for "work from home jobs."

The life we have chosen is not cheap; staying at home with my little loves and switching the entire financial burden to my husband is not feasible. I am an advanced practice registered nurse. I went back to school to help my family make more money. Turns out, all I did was increase my student loan debt. If nothing else, I have to work in order to pay for the education I thought would further my family. It has not. And I am sitting here, wallowing in the guilt of knowing that I have placed a huge financial burden on my husband's shoulders. We have five children, and working more than twenty-eight hours a week is something my heavy heart cannot handle.

I am battling silent killers: depression and anxiety. And I can get lost in them. Like I am now. All consumed by the panic, guilt, fear, and stress. My mind cannot stop running scenarios in which I lose my job and we lose our house. Trying to rationalize my situation is a full-time effort job. It is 8:36 a.m. and I am already exhausted, tearful, and empty. My eyes are burning and filling to the brim with invisible tears that refuse to spill over. I struggle daily, and when life throws me these curve balls it only heightens obsessive thoughts that trigger uncomfortable physical reactions. Oh, and did I mention that life throws me curve balls daily? I am a work-outside-the-home mom (when I can) of five kids who is struggling to keep her head above water as their needs change constantly. Who smiles her way through the day to acquaintances and strangers, coworkers and friends. But who breaks down every night in front of her husband and children.

Who cannot find the inner strength to fake happy within the four walls of her own home. I am someone trying to find a way to balance my chronic illness, the stigma attached to it, raise productive members of society, give my children the safety and love that I never feel, and keep our financial goals in mind. Did I mention that I battle a shopping fetish when I am placed under stress? Yeah, the extent to which my financial distress is related to that is probably astronomical. Trying to find productive coping mechanisms inside a mind that defaults to fear and negativity is also exhausting. Fighting the urges to fall into my spending habits, also exhausting. I am trying to make it, but for every two steps forward, I fall six steps back. I am like a gerbil on the wheel. I keep running and running only to be moving in circles. Making no progress and finding more doubt and discouragement than I care to admit.

I guess what I am saying here is that I want to talk about this. I want to share what living in darkness feels like. What searching for the light looks like. How to balance the black hole of depression with the light of Jesus. I do not feel happy. But I have gotten pretty good at faking it.

Intensive outpatient therapy, monthly counseling sessions and quarterly psychiatry appointments were all meant to armor me up for a battle that I have been and will be fighting until I die. It remains to be seen if my illness is terminal. What my prognosis is. Today, I would say the threat of succumbing to depression is high. Letting people down, unable to fulfill the expectations of work, placing the burden of being understaffed on my entire staff, makes me want out. Makes me think to myself that I cause too much heartache and turmoil. They would be better off with another employee, one who can go to work every day, maybe one without kids.

I find myself wondering why women thought it would be a good idea to protest all those years ago for the right to work outside the home. I cannot help but wonder if they gave me more choices or just more hurdles. I wonder what all the women who fought would think of me resenting their movement. I wonder if they are the ones to blame. Did they advocate having it all? Career, family, passion? Our society just is not set up that way. If you work, you are expected to make it a priority. For me, it is not. Staying afloat is. My husband's job comes first; he is better when he is employed. We have done the "husband laid off/wife working full time" thing and, to be honest, those were some of the most challenging times in our marriage. We were each filling roles that did not come naturally, and ones we did not want. These are not words that I can go around broadcasting. Social media would have my head.

Maybe you are finished with this book now that I have said it out loud, but there it is. I cannot fight against a system that says more stuff is better. I want the downsized lifestyle that would allow me to stay home. But that does not scream "accomplished" to people. I do not want to be accomplished; I want to be happy. It took us about six years to figure out how to find our balance. To accept it and not question it. To stop comparing our definition to everyone else's. But then, what happens is today: I have to call in to said place of employment because mom duty comes first, and my brain decides that every decision I have made up to this point is on the wrong side of the tracks.

Oh, hi anxiety, how ya doin'? Long time no see. Actually, you were just here last night, and the day before, and the day before. Like a torturous virus that refuses to grant my aching mind a reprieve. I am watching my three-year-old strategically place the cold cloth on her head where it hurts and craving an inner peace that I have yet to find.

If I have learned anything throughout this journey, it is that intrusive thoughts that are kept inside will break you down and destroy your capacity to cope. Speaking them aloud takes away their power and strengthens your resolve. It may not feel like it, but the world is better with you in it.

WHISHPERS

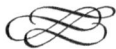

"**B**e safe out there," a gas station clerk told me recently as I paid for my desperately needed size-of-my-head coffee. Man, did I appreciate that sentiment. I am sure we all know it feels like the world is falling apart and crumbling. Every time we log onto our social media accounts, we are bombarded with shared links of tragedies happening all around us.

Some people listen for the whispers.

I tend to hear the loud voices that inundate my brain.

The same voices that told me I would never be worthy of another human's love.

The same voices that told me I would lose a child if I accepted Jesus as my Lord and Savior because he would want me to prove that I meant it when I said I believed.

I hear the loud voices, and then I turn inward and search for a whisper.

On some days, I just want to ignore the news outlets and pretend that we live in a world that sometimes does not scare me. But then I log onto my lovely social media accounts and am unfortunately reminded that is not the current climate.

I grew up with my sister and two brothers. Like most, I adore my siblings, but life has taken us into different directions; a few years ago, my baby brother came out to family, friends, and the world, as transgender.

I will leave her to tell her own story in her own time.

However, I would like to say that you cannot know how you feel about these topics until you experience them first-hand. Until you live in a world where those you love are being told they are unworthy or inadequate. You will not be able to understand the disheartening sense of Islamophobia until you fear for the life of a Muslim you love. You cannot form an opinion on transgender rights until someone you love begins transitioning. I guess you could, but it will change—because it is different when it is personal.

Me?

I have found myself spending a lot of time praying. Praying that they are safe. Praying that the world does not allow its fear to be a justification for its hatred.

In my experience, the world is not one that embraces diversity. Sure, everyone says how boring life would be if we were all the same, but I do not think they mean it.

It tells us to stop dreaming big and start living small. It encourages us to stop fighting against inequality and start accepting bias. It asks us to stop speaking up and standing out and persuades us to sit down and fit in.

I understand how easy it is for hateful speech to be broadcasted behind a computer screen, but I cannot accept it. We cannot wait for someone else to make a difference; we must hold each other accountable and *be* the difference.

Opinions are irrelevant; even if Muslims scare you and even if you believe a transgender individual has a mental illness. We must remember that *Golden Rule* we learned oh-so-long-ago but seem to have forgotten.

Treat others as you would want to be treated...

... online and in life.

I will continue on my quest of promoting kindness. I believe it matters. I will continue to live a life rooted in faith. A faith that encourages love, compassion, and respect. No, forget that. One that just encourages. I will continue to kneel in prayer and seek direction from The One who has given unconditional love and eternal life to my undeserving soul. I will continue cultivating my relationship with God, exploring his character and discerning his voice from the distraction the world seems so desperate to provide.

What I have learned is that, as a Christian, it is not my job to pass judgment. It is my job to quiet the noise and to glorify God in as many things as I can: in my words, in my actions, in my heart.

What I know to be true is that Jesus did not turn anyone away from his table.

And neither will I.

PART III

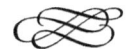

PART III
BALANCE AND BULLSHIRT

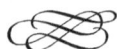

Oh, friends. Has mental health ever been so hard to navigate as it is in 2023? It seems like the world continues to be more complicated as we allow more and more electronic devices and technological advancements into our daily lives.

Enter social media. It is my Achilles heel. My kryptonite. My whatever makes a person go insane and waste time without being able to stop doing it. Addiction. I think the word I am looking for is addiction. I am addicted to social media.

I want to use it to change the world, but also, I cannot stop scrolling.

I want to use it to speak my truth, but also, I cannot stop reading the comment sections.

I want to use it to make people feel connected, but I cannot stop unfollowing all the influencers and celebrities who drive me batty.

It is so hard to balance the pros and cons of such apps. It is hard to find the value in them without also acknowledging the toxicity they breed.

Social media has been a thief of joy for me, and I struggle over whether I can cultivate enough positivity in my feeds to keep pouring energy into it. After all, we live in a world where everyone is online. Where everyone wants to have a platform, and where if you want to do anything you have to have a platform.

Living an offline life in an online world requires us to be mindful of our screen time.

The following pages are my thoughts on how to find balance within all of those complexities, and I can only hope that it allows you to cultivate an intentional relationship with your devices so you can be energized by your scrolling and not disheartened by it.

UN-SOCIAL MEDIA

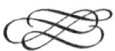

I have always been unsettled by technology. Okay, not always. Since about circa 2010, when I first was able to log in to Facebook from my QWERTY-capable slide phone.

Man, I am old.

Since then, I have been unsettled by technology and more specifically by social media, and to be even more specific: by Facebook and Instagram.

Over the last few years (and especially over the last few months), whenever I opened those apps on my phone, I thought to myself:

"What are you looking for?"

That is a tough question because I have not wanted to give an honest answer. I have had to spend a lot of time in reflection and meditation to candidly answer that question.

My gloss-over-the-facts, surface answers were: *"I'm just forming friendships and networking with other social media players"* or *"I'm just looking for funny memes because I could use some laughter"* or *"I am going to watch some mindless videos because I have had a long, hard day"* or *"I am going to be a good consumer and fellow blogger and support others I follow on social media."*

While I believe that was all true and potentially harmless, I'd step away from my phone (after having laughed my butt off and having left all the encouraging and supportive comments to boost my online friends in the algorithm) and I would feel as drained and empty as this iced coffee I am currently slurping through a straw while trying to get every last drop off each ice cube in the mug.

And then I would feel angry.

I was not rejuvenated and refreshed. I did not feel connected or productive. I did not feel anything that social media promised it would offer me if I gave it the things I could never get back: my time and my energy.

Step two was to really start acknowledging how I felt after mindlessly scrolling through the news feeds and again ask myself:

What are you looking for?

Okay, fine. I guess I am looking for a break. Because I would grab my phone when I was feeling stressed or overwhelmed. I used my index finger in a fluster to flick through the news feeds, absorbing hours of information in a matter of seconds—but here is the kicker: not processing it.

Predictably, I returned to the real world with a mind full of nonsense and anxiety from all the bad news and envy for other people's accomplishments without having done anything that filled my metaphorical cup, and I would find myself still needing an escape and not having an answer.

What are you looking for?

Here is where it got ugly, because I did not want to be this person. I did not like it or myself for thinking it, but if there is one thing I have learned through therapy and yoga it is to allow the thoughts to pass through you without judgment.

Here is what I was looking for:

I wanted a "big break". A viral post. A way to make money without having to leave my house. I was looking to prove that my writing was not for nothing. Because if my page had hundreds of thousands of followers or my videos had millions of views, then obviously I mattered more.

Cringe.

That brings us to step three and question two: *why did these things matter to me?*

Here it is, folks. The bottom line. I had been looking for acceptance and validity. I had been looking to prove to myself and my family and my friends and my fellow writers that I can be successful in this industry.

Success would mean that I have actual talent and that the trauma I have been through was meant for a larger purpose than just my own suffering. I had been looking to be a part of something bigger than myself, but in the process, I lost myself.

We truly have equated the internet's response with the validity of our story. The more tragic or unbelievable or obscene, the more shares and comments and responses; the more we are given the illusion of connecting through each other's pain when, really, it is just being used for mass entertainment and industry sales and follower fodder.

Here is a fact that I should feel embarrassed about but weirdly I do not: my last post on my Rebel Housewife blog had nine views.

Nine.

Views. Not even visitors.

If I am being honest, I probably accounted for three of

those views because if I am being even more honest—since why not tell all at this point—I like what I post.

I assume that by the standards of everyone in the industry, I am a big fat failure. My words have essentially reached no one. My story basically does not matter. To sum up: I am an idiot for exposing myself in this manner.

Let me digress for just a moment.

When I started my blog, I named it *Rebel Housewife* because I was rebelling against all the norms of what it meant to be a mom in a "*We have all-access to each other and therefore can compare ourselves to every other mother in the universe who had it together*" world. And I was calling nonsense because I knew the secret. The secret that no one has or had it together, and we should just be real and honest about that. We should not have to conform to invisible social media pressures.

You know the irony of it all? I did conform.

I put those with platforms on pedestals and aimed to be just like them.

The truth is not pretty, folks. But at least when we are honest with ourselves, we can make our decisions from a place of mindfulness and intention. We can give ourselves a choice. And that choice is: do we want to keep fading into the online lives of others, or do we want to be present in our own real lives?

Maybe for you the two are not mutually exclusive, but for me they are.

I have felt the nudge to pull away from social media for years. If you have been around me for any length of time, then you know I have done this back-and-forth dance before. I have deleted all the socials and committed to the blog but then got sucked back into the idea that having a social media following would mean a book deal and all the aforementioned perks of a big page.

The cycle would continue in this circular manner because I struggled with the fact that I was a hypocrite.

My shtick is about being more present and being online less, but still the goal has been for all y'all to spend more time on my social pages and extract an emotion from my words that would inevitably make you share my posts and comment on my pictures, and then the algorithm would find me relevant and I would grow.

The words have not exactly matched the intentions.

I have had to admit that I am addicted to my scrolling. I hate using the word addiction for something so many of us do, but just like I learned in middle school: just because everyone else is doing it, does not make it right.

Also, I feel this would be a good place to insert no judgment for everyone who finds actual and authentic joy in social media.

I did drop the socials for a while and I knew that likely meant I would never get an agent or a book deal. I spent a lot of time wrestling with those facts, but if I am going to be authentic then I have to believe that a New York Times bestseller does not validate my story.

It is not about the numbers.

It is about the impact.

I do not mean the impact that I could have on my readers. I mean the impact that I have on myself.

Writing fuels me. And when I am fueled, I am more present and more grateful. When I am those things, my family is the same. After all this time, the one thing I have come to realize is that the impact I have on my family (read: my kids) is really the most important one of all.

So here I am. Rebelling again. Telling the voice in my head that the viral stories are not marks of validation. That being published does not make my words mean more. That social media has not made me more social. Here I am, facing the ugly truth that those platforms suck my joy.

And I will not give another minute of my precious time and limited energy to anything other than that which brings me the absolute and purest form of joy.

I encourage you to do the same.

TROLL WHISPERER

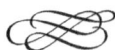

All right, this chapter is half serious and half giving a finger to the haters. I am going to go ahead and make it weird by doing a little Q&A about me by me.

Is everyone going to get on board with mental health? No.

Is everyone going to understand invisible illnesses? Of course not.

Does that bother me? If I am being honest, then yes. If I am being realistic, then no.

Am I really trying to change anyone's mind? No. Not because I do not want to, but because it is not possible.

I know this topic is going to bring about a knee-jerk reaction of *"but don't let it bother you,"* and *"the haters don't matter."* I know those reactions come from being uncomfortable in the unpleasant emotions. However, I want to encourage all of us to feel our distressing feelings. It is more than okay; it is necessary.

Avoiding our initial reaction is what takes us down those dark, winding, difficult to maneuver gravel roads. On the contrary, when we sit in the tension and allow ourselves (and each other) to acknowledge our pain, well, I think that is what promotes our inner peace and overall healing. It reminds us that we can trust our gut instincts. And we should use those instincts to explore our moral compasses and our personal values.

So that is what we are going to do with this interesting fact: the words I start out writing and the pieces I actually submit to be published are often very different pieces. To be honest (*and I am nothing if not honest*), this chapter was initially consumed by 'F' bombs followed by some harsh comparisons intertwined with immature insults. For no other reason than I was angry. Like chest-burning, adrenaline-pumping, bring-out-the-torches-to-set-some-things-on-fire angry. But anger is a secondary emotion. Meaning, I needed to peel away the layers and discover what was fueling the anger. I needed to bask in it and explore it and be honest in it, and then rephrase it.

Here is my toned-down rephrasing of the situation.

It turns out I am discouraged and hurt. It also turns out that anger is an easier expression of those uneasy, yet truthful, responses. You know, the ones that leave us feeling vulnerable because we admitted that something pierced through our ever-protective steel-like armor and rudely interrupted our fiercely sought-after calm.

Oh, context would be helpful. Such as what am I even talking about.

Okay. Here's the background story: I had a large publication repost one of my mental health pieces.

Insert all the *"I feel like a legit writer"* feels here.

I was absolutely grateful that they found enough value in my words *and* my story to share it on their website page. Now, I did have to tone it down and reword it slightly because of my tendency to be vulgar (*it is part of my charm*). But I think the heart of the piece remained intact.

Anyway, it was also shared on their social media pages, and of course the attention-seeking side of me got super excited, and I was like a dog sniffing out validation. I went and did the one thing I speak out against: I read the comments.

I know, I know. I am also an emotional masochist.

Overall, the comments seemed to be coming from other brave warriors who felt my pain and validated it by sharing their own. They responded from a place of love and support and empathy and I thought,

"It's not just me who struggles. It.is.not.just.me."

That is a powerful and intoxicating notion.

But then, of course, came the trolls. The ones who insert their opinion just to rile up the masses, and wouldn't you know it works. I got riled up.

There are all kinds of trolls that we know and love and have regrettably had the non-pleasure of interacting with. We have gotten sucked into their world and felt all the side effects of the emotional hurricane it stirs within us. So, before I get into the meat of the matter, let us explore the different kinds of trolls that exist on the internet.

The Arse Troll. Straight up arse-holes who are literally so mean that you know they are just there to stir a metaphorical pot. They are so ridiculous in their commentary that they do not even deserve the dignity of getting a response. Funnily enough, I find it easy to ignore them.

The Faux Supporter Troll. These are the ones who act like they are being supportive. Like they get you and what you are saying, but also they question if your experience was really that bad, and did it really warrant the feelings you felt? Ya know, they *know* someone who went through the same thing and *that* person they know had a different reaction. So *obvi* that is the *only* reaction that anyone in said situation will have ever in the world.

Ever.

The What Are You Even Saying Troll. These trolls are just circle talkers. They use big words in long sentences that seem like they sound good, but when strung together do not actually mean anything.

The Gaslighter Troll. They just come across all mean and ignorant. They go for the glory of the reaction. They want to provoke you with their commentary.

And it works.

You react.

And you respond.

And then they do not even understand why you are upset or why you felt the need to respond to them. They did not mean to imply what you think they implied. You should just ignore them in the same manner that you told them to ignore what they are commenting on.

It is not them; it is you.

The Toxic Masculinity Troll. These trolls. Insert *smh* here. They want everyone to "man up" and or "get over it." They want people to stop being so sensitive and to stop demanding respect. Like what kind of decent human being wants to be heard? They want everyone to bend over and take it because their egos are too fragile to handle the possibility that the problem is actually them.

Now, here is the thing. I know (*like am acutely aware of the fact*) that not everyone is going to give me a pat on the back for sharing my story. In fact, most people will not. After all, if most people *did* praise me for bringing awareness to mental health, then we would not need to be shattering any stigmas, would we?

Most of the time I do not know why I am writing. I do not know why I share things that are hard to share. I do not know if my teeny tiny online and community presence can actually make a difference. Maybe I just have an underlying need to be seen and *feel* seen. Maybe I am, in fact, an attention-seeking lady of the evening.

Or maybe I just think to myself that it would have been nice to know that people hurt the way I hurt. That they responded to trauma the way I responded. Maybe then I would not have spent twenty-three years of my life in the bitter dark pits of depression.

Every time I think the consequences of sharing my story outweigh the benefits, and I am ready to throw in the towel and say, *"Forget humanity,"* someone reaches out to me and gives me a thoughtful: *"Thank you for sharing said story."* Or they tell me: *"It would be a shame if you quit writing"* because, like it or not, words matter.

To be honest, I think they are the whispers; my angels in disguise and the ones that keep me going. It's interesting because if you expose yourself and you go viral, then you're brave—but if you expose yourself and it doesn't garner online acclaim, then bring on the pity and the "How could she talk about that?" But in the gathering of pity or those of us who "aren't going anywhere," there are a select few who will feel seen when they read or hear our story. Maybe even just one person will be on the other end of the screen or whatever communication method they are utilizing and they are worth it too.

One person is worth it.

Look, I am not here to please the masses or collect accolades (*despite my people-pleasing nature and my reaction to trolls*). I am here to share the story of how I have survived—and continue to survive—clinically diagnosed PTSD and clinically diagnosed persistent depressive disorder.

I was talking to a dear friend recently who said social media saved them. It brought awareness to issues they did not know were true medical issues. It has helped them to feel connected and more aware of treatment options.

My jaw hit the floor when they revealed this to me. Honestly, I had never considered that social media could be a positive place. I guess I figured it could have its positive moments, but I assumed overall we were all spending way too much emotional energy trying to be positive about the effects of online connection. I figured we *all* knew how ugly it was out there, but we were drawn to the drama anyway.

My friend's statement made me think (*as one does when given a point that one has never considered*) and wonder if *maybe* I have been too harsh to the online realm.

I really (*really, really*) do want social media to be a positive place where we can swap stories and trade encouraging words and connect with others who see the world as we see it. And maybe on a really (*really, really*) good day, it can give people the opportunity to understand us or, better yet, themselves.

We have gotten into this awful habit of saying that "*sticks and stones may break our bones but words will never hurt us*". The person who came up with that must have been the ultimate troll, and I call balderdash because words are some of the most powerful tools we have at our disposal. I mean, global power is accumulated by the *words* of world leaders, for God's sake. And I am just a wee bit sick of people reinforcing the false narrative that words do not matter. I think we would have less school bullies and online meanies if we just agreed that what we say *does* have an impact—and maybe we are not responsible for how people respond, but we *are* responsible for what we say.

That is a complicated concept to wrap a mind around, I know. It's a dialectical thought where two seemingly opposing ideas can be true at the same time, and those thoughts are gray and messy. I am learning that the collective 'we' find gray to be the most blinding color.

Maybe in the near future you will come across an article with a heading that gives you a strong emotional reaction. Maybe you go against your better judgment and read the comment section of said article. Maybe you will "see" trolls working overtime to tear down the people who can relate to the emotionally charged post. I would like to invite you ~~to kindly tell them to fuck off~~ to be an advocate for both the storytellers and the ones who connect with their narrative.

There is a person behind every story and every person (*and story*) matters.

Let people find *their* people. Let others express themselves without the fear of retaliation. Let people ask for help. *Start* equating reaching out for help with a beautiful and insatiable desire to live wholly and peacefully.

So, let us just be nicer about it. Especially online. Mmm-kay?

SUPERPOWERS

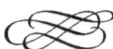

It turns out that I do comment on trending news topics more than I care to admit. It is such a fine line to not let political happenings infiltrate my inner peace while also fighting to secure a future I want my children to experience. In fact, where is the line between,

"I don't care about politics because it's all crooked," and

"Someone has to care because eventually this will impact me or my children or their children's children or their children's children." Okay, you get it.

To be honest, I have not found that line nor am I sure whether it even exists. I want to be mindful that I am just not another writer contributing to the already deafening noise because— I do not know if you have noticed—but it has been loud out here.

My way of straddling this impossibly thin line will be that I am *not* going to comment on the most recent global developments. That news and those pages have already monopolized all the media sites. To do you one better, I am not even going to provide my opinions on polarizing matters. I truly have to learn too much about all sides of all things and my feeble opinion would be a disservice to the magnitude of the topic.

However, I want to talk about the kind of emotions that are elicited when we talk about human rights. You know, emotions like anger and hatred and divisiveness. As we have seen over the last—what? Six years?—it can break up families and relationships. More than that, it can break people. I kind of think that when you take away people's options, you take away their hope.

Whoops. I inserted an opinion. But it is part of the point, so hang with me.

Losing hope. That is when it really hits the fan. Ultimately, I think that we are all casualties of a war based on political motivations and religious ideologies. It seems like we are losing control over what the world is doing to the collective "us." We can spend our emotional energy and precious time debating the value of what we *think* is happening, or we could explore how to *actually impact* what is happening.

I choose the latter.

Because I have been feeling the call to soften my heart, then I guess it would be prudent to mention that it does not matter which side of any debate you land on because, in my opinion, these suggestions are valuable to all sides (*since it seems we must take sides in all things, but I digress*).

Anyway, here are some actions we can take to help move us from social media activism to actual activism—if we are so inclined.

Money talks. Look, I run a non-profit. Awareness is great, but it does not pay the bills. If I am being completely honest, the hope in raising awareness is that it will lead to donations. As much as I wish it were not true, money makes the world go round. Money is power. So, put your money where your mouth is. Donate to organizations that line up with your theology. I cannot overstate this enough: if you *really* want to see change, you *got to* collect dem dollars.

Sign out. Stay out of the comment sections. No, seriously, log off. Do not read responses to emotionally charged posts out of curiosity. It will take you down a rabbit hole of emotional drama you cannot even see coming. I am serious. Stay off social media.

Okay, that is all well and good, but I am a realist. I reluctantly accept that social media is where everyone goes to share their everything, including their stinky opinions. So, if you *must* be involved in the online debates, then stick with accounts that are neutral and provide information on all ends of the spectrum. Feeding our minds with more of what we already fear, and worst-case scenarios will only increase our anxiety and our anger towards each other. On the flip side, feeding our minds with information and opinions that reinforce ours, well, that does the same. Branch out.

But not so much to be overcome with too many emotions.

Because when we are too overcome with emotion, we become too paralyzed to engage in productive ways to initiate change.

Reputation Matters. Dig in, friends. Like, get yourself a shovel and really go to town shoveling some dirt. What I mean is, do your research. Read reputable sites. Write down all your questions and then go looking for answers, and get your answers straight from the horse's mouth. Understand the system and the language, what it all means and what it is all saying, so that you can make an informed decision about how you can proceed with your impact. Do not go off the hype of other words or the emotions of social media posts. If you do not know what is happening in different countries and states and communities and why people are concerned about these situations, then look that up too. Don't formulate opinions off your BFF's shared meme. Find an actual, reputable news source and take it from them.

WWJD. This one is for my Christian friends. That is an acronym that dates back to my middle school days. Do we all still know what it stands for? I know it is weird to drop a handful of *F* bombs in a book and then launch into a spiel about Jesus. It seems that these types of situations all come down to our personal moral compass and value system. Let me tell you how many times I have found myself feeling righteous and committed to an ideology: so many that I did not even want to be around other people and the opinions that disagreed with what I *knew* to be right and true. I mean, my heart was convinced, and so I convicted e'rybody.

But over the last year or two, I have found myself being called to believe something greater, and that something greater is to love others fiercely.

I do that by listening. My gut reaction is still to bring out all my weapons of defense. And when I am ready to fire back with how the comment I just heard is an abomination to society, that is when I know it is time to pause.

And process.

And pray.

Believe it or not, it is always in the pauses and the prayers where I hear a soft whisper. It is a whisper that says something to the effect of *"Drop your righteousness and listen because what you're doing here is not creating a peaceful aura around you."* I kind of think that the Prince of Peace promotes peace, so you can draw your own conclusions there.

I invite you to go back and read scripture. Stop and pray for guidance. There is One who actually *knows* the outcome of this mess, and we spend so much of our faith thinking we *know* what he says that we forget to pause and listen to what he *actually* says.

If you slow down enough, I guarantee you will discover what your real role in the healing of this broken world entails, and I can almost *guarantee*, it will not be what you thought.

All right, y'all. I am sure there are more suggestions as to how we can transition our feelings from a sense of helplessness to acts of hopefulness. I know sometimes it seems like if we do not have the power to change everything, then what is the point in changing anything? Well, here is the point, dear friends:

It is only in the midst of the anything that we can end up changing everything.

Remember when the Supreme Court overturned Roe V. Wade? Did you see the meme circulating that said?

> "Scream.
> So that one day
> A hundred years from now
> Another sister will not have to
> Dry her tears wondering
> Where in history she lost her voice."

Every once in a while, something online will overwhelm me with its power. It will make me pause and it makes me think. Then I think some more and it ends up impacting me in a way that I want to honor.

So, I guess this story, this book, is my way of screaming. I want to encourage all those with falling tears that you *can* do something. It matters now and it *will* matter a hundred years from now.

STAYING IN LANES

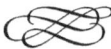

One time I told my counselor how I essentially fall off my rocker if I let too much time pass between therapy sessions, and she said that I am not the only one. She said that she likes to think of counseling as a dock that allows us to comfortably float in open waters.

We are all out floating on the sea or lake or ocean—or whatever body of water has a dock in it—and inevitably we will start running out of fuel. We need somewhere to land where the gas is plentiful and the ground is solid.

We make our way back to the dock—ideally before our tank of gas is empty—refuel with emotional acknowledgement and thought processing and coping mechanisms, and then we are ready to go back out into the open waters with enough stamina and supplies to keep us afloat.

That is basically a full-circle analogy to what I already thought counseling did for me and my brain. It was validating to hear that a therapist's view of counseling matches my own.

So, it is not just me and I am not alone.

I think ultimately that is the goal of everything that I put out into any writing space. To let all y'all know that you are not the only one and we are in this together.

Our humanity connects us.

At first, I think that sentiment can be hurtful. Especially when we are going through hard times, we are sure that we are going through the worst thing anyone has ever gone through and then someone comes up to us and says,

"Yeah, me too. I am going through that thing too. But it is worse and *here's how it's worse."*

That opens all the floodgates of emotion. We feel guilty that our smaller thing is impacting us more than their big thing. We feel ashamed that we shared our hard thing with someone going through a harder thing. We feel alone because we are not able to cope with whatever life is throwing at us when clearly there are worse things happening to other people who seem to be coping better.

And then we tell ourselves that our thing does not matter. It is not worth falling apart over. We bury it down deep inside of some pitch black *"it doesn't matter"* bottom of our stomach, and we keep our pain pushed so far down that it is hidden. Which only makes it grow because darkness begets darkness, and the only thing that can breach the dark is light. We are too ashamed to shed light on our hard thing, so it festers. As it festers, we continue to tell ourselves that it does not hurt as much as the thing is saying it hurts, so we do not try to heal from it. We keep our pain inside, not realizing how it is infil-trating every aspect of our lives and breaking us from the inside out.

I want to challenge this idea that suffering is a competition. That there are better awful things and worse awful things. That we can only be struggling if we are going through whatever we have deemed to be worse awful things, and anything less than awful should not be impacting us.

I am not sure who out there is making the lists of better awful, worse awful, horrific awful, and the continued spectrum of awful...

Actually, you know who I believe to be making the lists? Social media.

Our brains are flooded with stories of ultimate tragedies that do not even compare to our minimal struggles. We are constantly inundated in our scrolls with how it could be worse or how we should be grateful for what we have because our hard is not that hard compared to all the other trauma in the world. Maybe there is some truth to that. Maybe we should focus more on what we have going for us than going against us. But that fine line is difficult to balance, and I think the whole point is that we should not be comparing.

I came across a quote a few years ago that plays on repeat in my head when I start to think my pain is not worth processing.

"Trauma is trauma. Someone who drowns in seven inches of water is just as dead as someone who drowns in twenty feet of water."

People who do not feel their feelings or process their grief, however seemingly insignificant to the rest of the world's problems, end up being souls lost at sea. Drowning in open waters. Lacking a place to refuel and find rest.

They are people who end up being angry because they are hurting, and they are being told they are not hurting badly enough to warrant pain. And they become inconsiderate individuals who lack compassion and empathy because, well, if their pain does not matter, then why should anyone else's?

And instead of trying to heal ourselves, which we could do, we try to heal a whole wide world, which we cannot do.

So, I guess what I want to impart is this: It matters. Whatever *it* is. However big or small, in comparison to whatever you see in your news feed, it matters if it is hurting you.

Because you matter.

I want us all to consider: that which hurts us, hurts. Do not go trying to heal a broken world before you have healed your inner one. Acknowledge what you are feeling. Grieve when you feel loss. Cry when you feel pain. Celebrate when you feel joy.

We must allow ourselves to feel the entirety of the human experience. And we must give ourselves permission to respond to those feelings; in a healthy way.

Maybe, just maybe, *then* we will live in a world that is filled with less hurting people and more healing people. I will leave you with another quote since I am a quote person: *"Hurting people hurt people."*

So, maybe, just maybe, the opposite is true.

Maybe healing people heal people.

And maybe that ripples out to something bigger than online debates and social media commentary. Maybe it actually changes the world, one healing person at a time.

SOCIAL MEDIA SABBATICAL

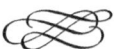

On Saturdays and Sundays, my social media feeds are full of all the events families are busy with while apparently having the time of their lives. We, however, were the family that purposefully kept our weekends quiet and free for as long as we could. There was a time when all of our littles were too little to partake in extracurricular activities and have sports they played. We kept our weekends free, not so we could make plans to run ourselves ragged; free so we could refill the empty buckets that our busy weeks drained dry in whatever way we wanted at that moment.

Sometimes that was in the form of sleeping in sans alarm clocks or waking up to watch the sunrise. We were free to stay in our pajamas all day or get dressed for a picnic in our favorite spot.

My kids could run around outside or lounge on the couch and watch television, and I could do laundry and yoga or nothing at all—and for a much too short forty-eight hours, the clock did not dictate our lives.

I used to feel bad about that until I realized that is how I like it, and our weekends were our sacred time together.

At the time I was worried my kids were missing out on team sports, but they ended up finding them at the right time.

One day, all too soon, my little ones will fly the coop and go their separate ways, and my house will not be full of laughing kids and messy floors. I will not be breaking up fights and telling them to go play somewhere else because we all need our space and privacy. The space between us will be far and wide; that is life, and we'll only have the memories of those precious weekends when we took the time to slow down and keep ourselves un-busy.

These moments were not social-media-picture worthy, but those days between the winding down of Fridays and the fresh start of Mondays were definitely our highlight reel.

My point here is that if that is you too, do not let the should-ing of staying busy diminish the magic-ness of resting.

Busy will find you. For as long as you can, stay un-busy.

It is not wasting time. It is basking in it.

SOCIAL DEADLY SINS

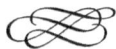

Sometimes it is hard to write about my opinion and my experiences without sounding like I am on a *"holier than thou"* rampage. But I guess that is technology in 2023 so, here we are.

Mental health and social media.

I feel like those two go together like oil and water, which is to say that they do not mix well at all. I do not remember always having a complicated relationship with social media. Truly, Myspace was fun and not all-encompassing. I think it started when our phones became mini portable computers, and everything had an app. I remember nursing my youngest son in the middle of the night and scrolling on my iPhone 3. I remember thinking that something was not quite right with that, but also I was trying to keep myself awake at one a.m., so what else was there to do? Since then, I have spent too much time and energy trying to incorporate social media into my life in a healthy way.

Where it enhances my life and does not detract from it.

I have had many a conflicted feeling. On the one hand, I

should be able to be on social media. Everyone else is and seems to enjoy it. It *should* be a positive force in my life. And on the other hand, if I have to try this hard to make something work for me, then it ain't working.

Here is where it gets a little high-horsey because now I am making a case for everyone in the entire universe to do the same. Actually, not really. I am not taking on any social media giants. I am pretty sure that dismantling the social media universe is impossible. But I think it is important that we acknowledge what it does to our minds and, inevitably, our lives.

I am just going to go full-on high horse and come at this from a spiritual perspective because that is what has been on my mind lately.

Ultimately, I feel like social media preys on all the seven deadly sins. You know the sins: gluttony and envy and greed and lust and pride and sloth and wrath. I feel like I do not need to elaborate on that because it is so "*duh.*" Or maybe it is so groundbreaking and revolutionary that I should delve into these thoughts in therapy.

The thing about the seven deadly sins is that they are alluring. I think we are drawn to them the way I am drawn to snacking when I am premenstrual. As such, when we are given an opportunity to indulge, we do. And when we indulge in those behaviors, it does feel good. For like a second. In the long run, we are all wondering, *"What did I even do today besides lie on the couch and binge-watch some grimy Netflix series?"*

We tell ourselves that we are staying informed and educating ourselves. Or we jump on some soap box and think that our words are making a difference in the world when, really, they just add to the noise.

For me, that is what social media does. It is so loud that I cannot hear anything except my own anxieties. I used to avoid quiet and rest like the plague. And what better way to keep myself distracted from my internal chaos than by grabbing my phone and scrolling? What I did not realize is that I was perpetuating the chaos rather than calming it.

Social media stole my mental health. I know that is a strong statement. That is also a statement that maybe sounds like a cop out; maybe also I *gave* social media my mental health. But the good news is that I reclaimed it. Since my mind is grateful, I am just going to go ahead and tell you what I filled my time with since I stopped scrolling every free moment and how that feels... mentally.

Yoga. I have been doing yoga so frequently and consistently that I daresay I am living yoga. And it is incredible. It is a practice that is so beautiful that I feel alive. And that is a feeling I used to avoid, but it turns out that feeling alive is a pretty fantastic way to live.

Writing. I have been writing consistently. And my brain thanks me for it. My thoughts are being processed and I do not feel weighed down by them. My mind is not jumbled and then becoming even more jumbled because instead of processing I am scrolling and adding to already overloaded synapses.

Meditation. Let me start by saying that meditation used to provoke panic attacks. And now it does not. And I think that is important to mention because I never thought that I would be able to meditate or find benefit in it. Instead, I distracted myself with, you guessed it, scrolling. But now I have taken to meditating and doing a 7 to 10-minute bedtime yoga practice, and my nervous system thanks me. I am learning to slow down and find beauty in the quiet rather than being afraid of it.

Faith. I am exploring my faith. I have started a read the

Bible in 52-weeks-type devotional, and something about having a higher power involved in my day just makes it better. I have felt called to actually read and study the Bible for quite a long time. But I never had time. Turns out that I had the time, I was just filling it with things that depleted me instead of the things that could fill me.

This is what it all comes down to: scrolling takes time.

And brain power.

And mental energy.

And it makes us think that we are busier and more in trouble than we actually are. It lies to us and tells us that we do not have time to do things that will make us better. I kind of think that people who do not have time to make themselves better are easier to control. It's easier to feed divisive and painful information to them. It's easier to paralyze the masses because they are so focused on their screens that they are not looking up to see what is really happening.

And now I went full-on conspiracy theorist. That took an unexpected turn.

I mean, I do not think that social media was invented as a mind control for the masses. But I kind of think that is what it has turned into. So, here is my actual, ultimate point:

Stop.

Notice.

Log off.

Live.

Look up every once in a while, so that you can take stock of what you are filling your time and your mind with, and then ask yourself: *Is this what I want to fill my time and mind with?*

Because maybe we all get so lost in the noise that we forget how beautiful and fulfilling it can be to slow down in the quiet.

SMOKING GUN

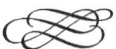

I am going to use an analogy here, and the analogy is between cigarettes and social media. I know it sounds like it is going to be weird, but I *think* that it is going to make sense. Bear with me as I fumble through this one and start with, you guessed it, a quick backstory:

I used to ask my patients, *"Are you interested in quitting smoking?"*

They almost always responded with a resounding: *"Of course I'm interested!"*

Then I would jump right to how we could help make that happen, and almost always I saw a look of panic crossing their faces followed by a *"Oh, I'm not ready to quit"* response. And for the longest time, I was confused.

What is the difference?

Who is interested but not ready? Aren't the two synonyms?

Au contraire.

How many of us are interested in things but not ready to take the leap? Dare I say all of us? Okay, I will not use an absolute like "all of us," but I will say (*probably*) many of us are. Aren't we interested in advancing our careers, or taking a leap into that relationship we have been hoping for, or pursuing our passions and living out our dreams?

I think so.

But are we *ready* to take the steps and make the sacrifices to do it?

Ummmm... I think that is a different beast altogether.

So now, when I talk to patients, I ask a different question: *"Are you ready to quit smoking?"* To be honest, I get so many *"nos"* and *"not yets"* that when someone says *"yes"* I am almost always taken aback and need a minute to gather my thoughts and concoct a coherent follow up sentence that will be helpful in their smoking cessation journey.

Here is where the analogy comes in. I have kind of an unconventional belief that social media is the same as a nicotine (*or really any*) addiction, with one minor but major difference. Nicotine dependence and addiction are recognized as medical conditions. They are actual diagnoses.

I did a quick Google search to see if social media addiction is a recognized medical condition and, surprise, surprise Google says it is not.

Yet.

I know it is not popular to say that social media is an addiction and that we are almost all addicted, but when I look at what an addiction is, I cannot help but notice way too many similarities between my nicotine-dependent friends and my social media ones. I could launch into a *"Webster defines addiction as..."* speech here, but to be honest that kind of lingo bores me. Instead, I am going to launch into what I believe to be facts about addiction, so **disclaimer time: these might be opin-**

ions; I am going off my own knowledge base and experi-
ence here.

- We turn to something to help make ourselves feel happier.
- We turn to something to help ourselves alleviate stress.
- We find ourselves turning to it absentmindedly and being under its influence without even realizing it.
- We feel lost without it.
- We feel a high when we are under its influence, and we chase that high like motherfucking champs.
- We explain why we are in control over the thing we turn to and how it does not actually have any power over us.
- We rationalize away the ways in which we know it to be destructive.
- We tell ourselves that we could stop if we really wanted to, but we do not really want to.
- We know the consequences of the thing and how it negatively impacts us, but the high is too high for us to let go of.

Even though I am ending that last sentence-slash-point in a preposition, my point is that I think we are with social media where we were with smoking in the forties (*1940s, that is*): It is cool, and everyone's doing it. But thirty-five years from now, when everyone is riddled with dopamine burnouts, suicidal ideations, and debilitating anxiety disorders, maybe we will realize that we need to quit that which kills us.

That kind of sounds harsh and dramatic, but here is where I

am circling back to my smoking analogy: I talk to so many people who are *interested* in getting off social media. But they are not actually *ready* to get off social media. When I tell people I am not on social media *(because many people want me to find out a lot of pertinent societal information via social media)* and I have to launch into the spiel of *"Oh, well, I'm not on social media,"* and then they are all like, *"Wait, you are not on social media? That is so good, I wish I could do that, but I am not really on it that much"* or *"I know, it really makes me feel sad-slash-it's the downfall of society, but I like to see people's pictures and keep up with my friends."*

Man, do I get that.

I rationalized the faux benefits of social media for fifteen years. And let me tell you what is happening inside me right now. I am coming up on six months of social media sobriety. One might think that makes it easier to be off all the apps.

Not so.

Where I am now gives me enough distance from thinking that I can manage it again. That I can just get on and scroll as long as I set up boundaries and follow them. I am wondering what I am missing and am sure that I am missing something. The FOMO is running rampant. Especially as my kids are becoming more involved with peers. I *need* to Facebook-stalk.

Like I am withdrawing from a toxic substance, and it is beckoning me to return to it.

I am almost actively fighting the urge to not log back into my Instagram and Facebook. It is just a quick username and password to reactivate, and then I can feel a sigh of relief as I scroll and stalk and do all the social media things that make the world go round. I keep thinking that there are some perks to social media, and that it did not really make me feel as bad as I thought it did, and that I can control it from here on out because I just needed a break.

WAS I NOT SUPPOSED TO SAY THAT?

Man, addiction messes with your head.

Here is what I know to be true: I was not reading books when I was on social media because I did not have time because I spent more time than I realized scrolling. In fact, I thought I hated reading books, but it turns out they can be pretty exhilarating—and seeing words on a page and then thinking and reflecting on those words and ideas is actually pretty incredible.

I was not journaling, and my head was so full of clutter that I could not think straight. I was not writing regularly, and my heart ached to do so. I was not working my way through the Bible and working on developing a relationship with God for the first time ever and realizing *that* is where actual fulfillment and enlightenment lies.

And here is the kicker: I was not keeping up with friends. At least not in a productive way. I think I was judging them and feeling envious of them. I was ready to move on from them because their posts would be so infuriating to me. I think social media cost me more friends than it kept. I think I forgot how to listen, and I forgot how to be compassionate. I did not even know it was happening, as I was consumed by self-righteous thoughts being reinforced by all the pages I followed with similar beliefs.

Bottom line: I was more distracted and more anxious and more judgmental when I was on social media.

And then there's the whole setting boundaries thing. Been there done that. I've tried the *"I'll only go on for an hour in the morning and then stay off the rest of the day"* type thing, only for my fingers to find their way to my app. I'd open it and scroll real quick, just to see if anything had been updated since I'd last checked since obviously all life-altering events are happening on social media, and then my brain would be clogged and sleepy, I was crabby and I felt guilt for crossing my own self-made boundaries.

What kind of human cannot even maintain a boundary that they have set?

That is what makes me feel (*even more*) like social media is an addiction. When you cannot dabble in it. When you cannot maintain boundaries. When you think you have control but are really being controlled by it. That happens because brain chemicals are being altered or because minds are being held hostage by an alternate reality.

The truth is that we really try to escape from our problems, and social media is that outlet. But really, I think we need to escape *from* social media. Or at least be conscious of how it is impacting us. I think we need to move from denial into awareness.

Back to my cigarette analogy: smokers *know* what can happen if they keep smoking. It is not a mystery. Increased risk of cancer and lung disease and heart disease—they know. Not one of my patients has ever been surprised to hear me tell them the consequences of persistent smoking.

They choose smoking anyway.

I just think that we need to acknowledge how social media might be impacting our mental health and our real life relationships and our mood and our ability to enjoy a life outside of screens. How it is stealing our time and eliminating our joy. How it is wasting our present moments and leaving us feeling lonely and alone.

Then we can decide, purposefully, if we are going to choose it anyway.

LOG OFF MORE

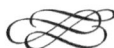

These past few, well, years, I have been thinking about social media and what it means to try to be a whatever I am trying to be online, and to have some sort of success it seems an account needs to have one or two or all of the following:

(Before we start, let me insert a "no judgment" disclaimer to any who run their accounts using the following techniques, as those accounts are smart and business savvy and successful, and probably producing an income—and I am none of the above.)

Back to what large following accounts seem to have in common based solely on my observations:

1. Controversial posts asking controversial questions to get engagement.
2. Ridiculous posts that make you go "whhhhhhhhy would someone do this" and the answer is to get shares.

3. Opinionated posts to provoke an anti-opinion from followers and thereby increase visibility in the algorithms.
4. Large scale home renovations with all the updates because if we are not envious of all the things they can do that we cannot, why are we even following them?
5. Fancy schmancy vacations and all the moments via stories because, again, if your jealousy is not seething, then how are they going to keep us buying what they are selling?
6. That elusive wow factor that just draws people in. I do not even know what the wow factor is, I just know that I do not have it.
7. Posts telling people what they are doing wrong and why they need said account to do it right.
8. Posts telling people that the way to afford home renovations and fancy vacations and extravagant lifestyles is to buy what they are selling in the form of a business or course of some kind.

I know what you are thinking: I am jealous because they have it and I do not, and I am here to say that is only about 67% accurate.

You see, all of the above is meant to keep our noses buried in our phones and our debit cards in our hands and our yearnings close and our actual experiences far.

That, friend, is why my online presence is small and intimate. No, I am not saying that I am better than the other accounts, or that I am a diamond in the rough, or that I can give you something the other accounts cannot.

I am just saying I do not want to play the game.

Honestly, I have dabbled in the game. I have tried to squeeze my way off the bench and onto the field, but, y'all, I suck at this game.

I am not interested in jumping on the trendiest news topics unless they are human-rights related and I just think that equality is worth my voice; I am not interested in sharing what my family does or where we go because, honestly, I am more focused on living the moments with them than trying to invoke a sense of FOMO behind a screen to keep followers coming back for more. If I am being 100 percent honest, I also have an intense-perhaps irrational- fear of stalkers and kidnappers so I would rather keep family outings as private as possible.

I do not want you to buy anything from me except my writing because I am hypocritical like that.

Truthfully, what I hope you find here is a reminder that my work does not deserve all your attention, or all your efforts, and you certainly will not feel rested or connected by trying to keep up with the social medias.

By all means, budget time to scroll your feeds if you enjoy it, and budget money to support your favorite influencers if it fills you up, but my online spaces are just a friendly reminder that you don't actually need what anyone is selling and if we keep our heads buried in our screens, then we are missing out on life. My only point here is to tell you that you don't need to be online.

You are not falling behind in life.

You are not missing out on any news.

Enjoy the silence.

Enjoy the nothing.

Enjoy the space between what has to be done and what can wait.

Everything else on social media platforms is an illusion to keep you chasing after things that will never fill you up.

You will find your real joy in your real life so go and live it.

LET IT BE

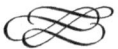

I want to write something profound and brilliant.

I want to knock your socks off with an inspirational mantra.

I want to blow your mind with an insight so deep it makes you rethink everything you have ever thought.

But all I can think to say is this:

I am exhausted.

Tapped out.

But also, I feel amazing. Like my body is finally my home and my mood is finally elevated enough to function without threatening to destroy the light I am gaining.

But also, I am over it, and I want so many things to be done and I want to move on and I want things to change.

I want to be amazing, but also I just want to be me.

My brain and the insides of my eye sockets feel like they could hibernate for a few winters before they, once again, become fully functioning.

I do not really know what to do with any of that, and I am processing these opposite-spectrum emotions and learning how to navigate dreams and desires and responsibilities in a world where I am both depleted and energized; tired and alive.

Where I have small numbers and little clout, but big dreams and unlimited desire.

I do not even think I have a point here, except to say that it is okay if you are all the things.

It is okay if you are a feeling person in a confusing world.

I think what I really want to say is forget this skewed world that equates success with large numbers and high dollars.

It is okay if you never take your passions and turn them into profit, and you are brave for exploring your limits even if no one says it.

Do all the things with purpose or do nothing at all with joy, and just know that your existence is magnificent even if your post likes are minimal.

It is not the numbers that determine your value, nor is your value determined by how many people see you or praise you or cheer you on. It is not determined by how much you do or what you accomplish.

I find the best people are the unnoticed and the underrated.

All that matters is that we do what we do with kindness and authenticity and love.

Keep going, friends.

Even if no one is watching.

Scratch that.

Especially when no one is watching.

HAPPY HAPPY JOY JOY

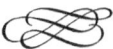

Things have been heavy over the last... I want to say three years, but I think it has really been heavily hitting the fan since 2016, hasn't it? I mean, not just from a personal standpoint, but from a global one.

It is not enough that we have been battling pandemics and politics for the last several years, but throw in wars and mass shootings and it is pretty easy to get swallowed up whole in grief and despair.

But who can function there?

Or perhaps more accurately, who *wants* to function there?

I do not know about you, but when I get caught up in the heavy of it all, I tend to become overwhelmed and overstimulated, and if y'all know anything about anxiety, those are pretty much two major precursors to a panic attack. To be honest, my spirit is slightly worn out, and continuing the conversation about things like common-sense gun laws and women's rights to their own bodies would be a disservice to my own mental health. (Let me go ahead and insert here that these issues are not all inclusive and should not be taken to mean that these are the only conversations of value).

Which always leads me back to the question: can we care and advocate for change and still be allowed to rest?

Yes, friends. Yes, we can. I am not a fan of should-ing on ourselves, *but* rest is a should.

These issues are not a sprint to the finish line. The problems were not created overnight, and the solutions will not be found in an instant. It is more like a marathon. It is going to take time and for us to go the distance and see it through, we *have* to find our strength. We *have* to feed our souls. I think that seemingly impossible stamina is found in rest and reflection.

I have started referring to that as 'pockets of joy.' It makes me feel less guilty for finding happy when my scrolling is filled with tragedy and my soul is filled with fear. My counselor tells me that guilt is reserved for those who have done something wrong, and I have to remind myself of that often.

Joy is not wrong.

In fact, it is necessary, and it is life-giving and it feeds our passions and desires for better. It is a mandatory balance in a world that has so much sad. All that to say that I had a pretty pure pocket of joy this past weekend which I want to share with you. Not in a *"look at me"* kind of way, but in a *"there is still so much beauty in the world, and I will not let it pass me by without acknowledging it"* kind of way.

I am going to begin by setting the scene so,

Without further ado...

It started with the absolute most gorgeous morning. I mean crystal clear, deep-blue skies with a few puffy, brilliantly white clouds scattered throughout. An actual painting.

And the weather: insert chef's kiss here because it was

fantastic. Picture the perfect amount of breeze that moves just enough air to keep stagnant energy from collecting around your personal space. It was like a Goldilocks situation because it was not too hot, and it was not too cold. It was just right.

It was one of those mornings when I could sit outside and be completely comfortable in lightweight cotton pajamas. I did not need a fan or a blanket. I could drink my hot coffee without profusely sweating, and it was okay when it cooled off since I was not relying on it to warm up my insides.

I literally live all year long for mornings like this one. I am the kind of person who soaks up all that glory in solitude and then, when my spirit is satisfied, I drag all my people out to experience it with me.

So I forced my husband to sip the coffee I persuaded him to make (*because gorgeous mornings start with coffee even when you do not drink coffee*) outside in one of our white peeling-paint, armrest-broken-off rocking chairs. And I brought out the dog because she loves some fresh air, and all the spawn who woke up before noon because they need some fresh air.

As we sat on the porch, our #3 and #4 kicked a soccer ball all through the front yard and ran after it. The thing about kids running is that they look absolutely free. When I run, I feel like my joints are getting crushed beneath the weight of my nearly forty-year-old body. It seems like my ankles could buckle and I would easily be thrown forward on my face from the inertia of it all. I feel like a herd of elephants traipsing through the yard as my feet drag under me. Like do they even rise from the ground or are they too dense to do so? It is the opposite of whatever "carefree" looks like.

But when my kids run, man, they are light. Almost hopping through the air, feet barely tapping the ground for stability. The wind blows through their hair and passes through their clothes, and it does not even slow them down. I do not think their breath quickens. God, I absolutely love to watch my kids run.

Then there was our dog. Lying in the grass, looking calm and cool and collected. My kids are truly her pups, and I think she felt the same freedom in their presence and was just taking it all in alongside me.

I looked over at my husband and I said, "*You know what, we actually dreamed about this moment. We actually dreamed about sitting on a front porch, drinking coffee while our kids ran around in our front yard, free from traffic and people, and having a dog lying in the freshly cut grass alongside us.*"

In that moment, in that realization, I felt actual joy. Pure, unadulterated joy. "*Isn't that amazing?*"

This is not me saying, "*Oh we're living our dreams*" as in, "*We are living our best life*" kind of way. I say that in a "*Most of the time it feels like we aren't*" kind of way.

Let me just fill you in on a few little tidbits to really drive the point home.

We are still as middle class as they come. Every time we think we will make headway in our finances, a car craps out or a kid ends up in the emergency room. And when we think we will be able to pay off the most recent catastrophe, we are met head-on by a new one, like broken appliances or PTO-less days off work because of sick kids. Is it just me, or can the PTO not keep up with the number of sick days required to parent these days? But I digress.

Our house looks like an actual battlefield with broken curtain rods in our living room that are curved in places where curtain rods do not normally bend, but they still keep the fabric off the ground, so they will do. We have so many holes in our walls from kids opening doors in a way that makes me wonder why we waste money on door stops, and did the person who invented said door stops even have kids? There are actual metal studs showing on the corners of our walls because I have no fucking clue why. Our broken blinds are covered in teeth marks from the dog who cannot open them but still wants to see out.

We have dreams of taking our kids to Disney World, and our kids have dreams of getting on an airplane. We would love to hop in an RV and drive all across the country on a whim. A 'parent's only' vacation is on the bucket list, and I would give my one working coffee maker to find a way to make this writing gig prosperous.

Truth be told, there are times when I feel so selfish for having brought kids into this world. I mean, they are amazing humans and I think they are the best part of every day. But maybe I should have more seriously considered whether I wanted them to have to fight these fights and face their own personal demons on top of all the other tragedies the world unleashes on the daily.

But then mornings like this happen, and I watch them run —and I want them to feel that sense of genuine joy. The kind of joy that can only come from doing absolutely nothing in the midst of an ordinary Sunday morning.

It is pretty incredible that in the middle of all the chaos and worldly terror and absolute uncertainty all around, in that moment I felt *actual joy*. And that joy, man... It was almost like I experienced a sigh of relief, and with that release came an ache and understanding that *this* is what it is all about. It was almost like all the other things were not happening. It was almost like discovering that it is all going to be okay.

Not just because it is going to be okay. It is going to be okay because we are going to invest our time and energy into making the wrongs we see in the world... right. We can only do that when we fill ourselves with permission to slow down and acknowledge that it is all about moments and then take some time to delight in them.

When the world feels as heavy as it has and we start to get in our heads about how it is all falling apart, I think it is important to remember a few things. We can feel the heavy and not be consumed by it. We can look for pockets of joy and bask in them. We can care about the injustices in the world and continue to live our lives. We can fight for change and still take time to rest.

Dialectical thinking at its finest, eh?

I will end these ramblings with an invitation, if you will.

Let us fight when we are rejuvenated and rest when we are not. Let us allow ourselves to grieve when we feel sad and to feel joy when it finds us. Even if the world or *our world* is falling apart. Let us not feel the need to qualify the joy or rationalize the joy or feel guilty for the joy. Because the more I think about it, the more I think that joy is just hope on steroids.

And, uh, if there is one thing I think the world needs more of, it is hope.

DEAR DIARY

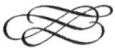

O nce upon a time I was off social media for twenty-seven days now.

Like, off, off.

Like, "not even logging in to check something really quick" off.

Which is approximately twenty-seven days after I claimed I was getting off social media. I guess I would say I had to taper off the socials. I mean give or take because it is not like I have been ticking off the days on a calendar. It might sound dramatic, but I feel like I am in recovery. That I am an addict who is 27 days sober and living clean.

We do not do that usually. We do not put social media in the same category as other addictions.

Do we?

There are alcoholics and drug addicts and cigarette smokers. Those who reach for their substance of choice whenever life becomes too much, and they need an outlet or a distraction.

We do not do that with social media, though we do reach

for it when we need a distraction or an escape; though we are chasing the dopamine high of post likes and notifications; though it removes us from what is happening right in front of us, and we are glad that it does.

One recent lazy Sunday afternoon, my husband was scrolling through our streaming apps and settled on rewatching *The Matrix*. As the movie played, I thought to myself that at one point in my life—you know, the first fifty times I saw it—this movie seemed completely absurd. People engulfed by machines. Living a faux life and having no concept of reality.

This time it hit differently.

I thought, "*Holy moly. It's happening.*"

I know I know I know but hang with me.

Maybe not in the theatrical Hollywood way that the movie portrayed, of robots consuming humans as energy sources, but kind of.

We are absolutely consumed by what is happening on our screens, and we are absolutely unaware of what is real.

We are being fed what to think and how to feel by these applications without even realizing the influence we are under.

We have the ability to feel the world's atrocities in a split second and we just are not capable of processing that, so instead we lash out at each other. Sow discord and division through the guise of sharing information meant to give us an emotional reaction. And the thing about humans is, we are emotional, we will react, and usually when we react from an emotional standpoint, we do not react kindly.

So here I am. Twenty-seven days sober. Calling a spade a spade. In recovery from an addiction that was ripping me apart from the inside.

Those twenty-seven days I thought about so many

wonderful things. Such as how beautiful the leaves are as they turn from their shades of yellow to burnt orange and fiery red. I thought about how wonderful it is to feel my children's heartbeat against my chest when they come up to hug me and I soaked it in.

Undistracted.

I read the funniest, wittiest book and enjoyed it. Me. Liking reading. Weird.

I have been working through a devotional, and I have been journaling, and I have been listening to my body and what it needs.

And I have been responding.

I have decluttered my brain.

Don't get me wrong: it has been as nutty as a Nutter Butter around here. We have had sick kids and car breakdowns and teenage angst and all the things that reap stress and chaos, but here is the kicker.

I am okay.

With the space I need to manage the things happening right in front of me. And to do it with joy.

And it feels amazing.

I have done absolutely nothing impressive, and yet I have felt absolutely remarkable.

I feel like I have woken up and been given a chance to soak in the beauty of life.

I always say that time moves too fast and I cannot grasp it, and it is slipping through my fingers, but getting off social media has freed up—oh, I do not know—four hours a day of my life. And that is probably a conservative estimate. I do not even want to know the time I actually spent online. I am not that sober.

It is amazing how much life can be lived and felt and appreciated when you are not scrolling for some four-odd hours a day.

You are rolling your eyes, aren't you?

I can feel you rolling your eyes at me.

I know, because I used to do the same.

I had social media under control, and honest to goodness believed it was not controlling me.

But that is the thing with addiction. We do not see it until we step away from it.

Twenty-seven days sober.

Counting every minute and soaking up every second of having woken up to being given the one thing I always begged for more...

... time.

AN INVITATION

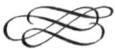

M y sister said the most brilliant thing to me, and I must share:

"Are you solving the problem or are you creating a new one?"

Every single one of us should pause and ask ourselves this as we fight for the causes that speak to our souls.

Are we fixing the problem or are we making it worse?

Right hand to God, that's genius.

So, as I lose all respect for even mentioning the words *politics* and *common sense* in the same sentence, here is my invitation:

Really reflect on that statement as you take to your social media platforms and profiles and post information (or misinformation) about politically charged topics.

Let that statement soak in as you react to news in the world and take to organizing protests and participating in sit-ins.

What are you helping?

Who are you hurting?

Just an invitation to make an informed decision before you try changing the world and its ways.

In doing so, I bet what you will find is that change does not always need to happen out in the world; it needs to happen within our own selves.

Changing ourselves.

Self-control and awareness.

Mindfulness.

That is how we change the world.

PART IV

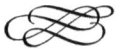

PART IV
LOVE LETTERS

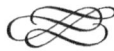

These "chapters" are for you, friends.

Love letters.

Reminders.

We can strive to be our best selves on the daily, but our "as is" selves are awfully great too.

Keep going.

Keep peeling.

Keep healing.

After all you have been through, there is joy that is waiting for you.

DEAR MOM-BOD

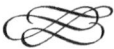

D ear Mom-Bod,

Somewhere between growing humans and birthing them, our baby bumps go from "She looks so cute!" to "She let herself go."

For some reason, we are conditioned to believe that our postpartum bodies should reflect our pre-partum selves. We are encouraged to erase all physical signs that we have been transformed literally from the inside out.

Let me assure you that no amount of crunches or Kegels will take a mom of five's belly back to her college belly, and let me assure you that there is nothing wrong with that.

Sure, we may live in a world that offers more serums, creams, and gym memberships than it does mind, body, and spirit connections, but our worth is not measured by the degree to which we can eliminate all outer signs of our transformation.

There is more to this journey than maintaining the illusion of youth on our faces and perfection in our bodies.

Healing from trauma, working towards inner peace and finding our breath in the chaos offers just as much confidence as six-pack abs and wrinkle-free faces—maybe more.

My point is that your body is strong and capable and beautiful in its "as is" condition. Some bodies are toned and some are squishy, but your body tells a story—and that story matters.

Love, Me

DEAR LEARNING YOUR VALUE

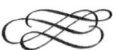

D ear Learning Your Value,

Someone asked me recently if I have to fill in my brows or if they are just heavy on their own. It was within the context of the conversation, so it was not weird—but leave it to me to struggle to keep it not weird.

My brain wanted to answer with a "Nope, big brows and big noses go together," but I have learned not to say anything about my nose. It puts people in an awkward position. They are not quite sure if they should laugh because they are not quite sure if I am joking since this schnoz is, in fact, large.

I grew up in a time where taking up space was not as celebrated as it is now, and if you are thinking, "Well, Sara, it's not really celebrated now," then that is even more to my point.

Small. Dainty. Petite.

Fitting into spaces and not taking them up.

That is what you should want.

A nose with "character" (that is what people say when they want to be tactful about what is happening here) brought on lots of teasing and pity. I often felt that when I walked into a room I was a nose on a neck, and that I needed to do something about that.

It was not until my husband told me he liked my nose (cue in all the "awwws") and I saw it on my daughter's face (and her face is absolutely beautiful) that I started coming to terms with this thang.

You know how sometimes you meet people and you are like, "Meh, they're all-right looking," but then you get to know them and you're like, "Oh, wow, you're really attractive"? I have been thinking that is what has been happening with me on this self-acceptance journey.

I am working really hard to be a person that I like because I am with myself all day, every day, and since I cannot escape that fact, I may as well cultivate a human that I enjoy being around.

And it turns out the more I practice liking myself, the more I like what is on my face. To be honest, we are friends now.

The point here is that if you happen to like what you got going on—even if it draws negative attention because it does not fit in the box of whatever beauty standards we are following now—then I invite you to spend some time getting to know the person behind it. I bet that person is the bee's knees and deserves to take up as much space as they want.

Scratch that; I KNOW it.

Love, Me

DEAR HELPER

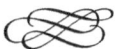

D ear Helper,

I have never been good at absolutes, like getting on my mat every morning. I can usually talk myself out of things that make me feel better by convincing myself I need to rest. I'm not going to lie, it's been difficult to discern whether I need rest or if my depression is keeping me low.

About twelve years ago, I stopped eating fast food. Not for my cholesterol or body image, but because eating it made me so violently ill that it just was not worth it.

Up until about five years ago, I enjoyed a weekly chocolate Long John (okay, biweekly because both hump day and Fri-yay deserve celebratory donuts) from QT, and side note: they really have the best donuts. Anyway, I stopped eating them because the post-pastry mental and physical lull just was not worth it.

I am not good at being proactive towards my mental health, but I am learning that I am pretty good at being preventive against my mental illness. It sounds like those are the same, but turns out that perspective is everything.

It does not really feel good to drag myself out of bed before dawn, slap on some leggings, pull out the mat, and move my body. But it feels worse to be tense all day, lack patience with my family, and feel easily overwhelmed by mundane tasks.

All that to say, sometimes we will find more motivation in avoiding consequences than in reaping benefits.

Perhaps you are avoiding the thing because it is just too much, but in those moments it helps to pause and ask yourself: are you finding peace in the avoidance or is it just leading to further despair?

If it is the latter, you know what to do, my friends. Do the dang thang. Your present self may not be on board, but your future self will thank you.

I know we want to do the right thing for what we think is the right reason, but not wanting to be lost in darkness is a good enough reason. And while we may strive to be more present, sometimes we have to consider what groundwork we are laying for tomorrow.

It may not be easy to recognize what is helping us, but if we allow ourselves a moment to pause, breathe, and notice, we can recognize what is harming us.

And in responding to that, we are able to help ourselves.

Love, Me

DEAR TRYING TO HEAL

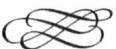

D ear Trying to Heal,

Just recently, I was telling my ol' faithful how I'm confusing myself. I feel like two different people. Half of me is content, confident, hopeful, optimistic, and did I mention content?

The other side of me is just... I do not know how to really capture it other than to say sad. Not in a depression way and not meaning that anything bad is happening. Just in a way that says: there is sadness with a side of heavy, and let us not forget fear, and I feel its presence.

He responded with: "Which side are you feeding?"

In case you do not know, that is a reference to one of my all-time favorite memes. I think it is based on a proverb, but I am not sophisticated enough to quote anything other than internet memes.

Anyway.

It is a story about a grandfather telling his grandson how

there are two wolves inside all of us. Essentially, one of the wolves represents goodness and the other represents pain. The grandson asks his grandfather which wolf wins? And he responds with: "The one you feed."

Mind blowing, right?

If I am being honest, I think I am feeding into the sadness. Call it a spiritual battle or just a mental default to pessimism, but I lean into sad more than content. In my defense, content is harder. I do not know why all things that bring joy require us to put forth so much time and energy and effort?

Like how amazing would it be if binge-watching *The Good Place* on repeat, lounging on the couch eating pizza and ice cream at all hours of the day, and scrolling endlessly on our phones brought us more than a temporary high? Why is it that the things that are easy actually make things hard?

Anyway.

My point here is now that I have been made acutely aware that the wolf I am feeding is not my friend, and since he is a liar I have decided to lean into truth so that I not only find my peace but keep it, and I just want to encourage you to do the same.

Log off.

Pause.

Close your eyes.

Breathe.

Notice.

Now is as good a time as any to turn your partial pain into complete healing. It will not be easy. In fact, it will be really hard. But keep going because present-you deserves a future-you who is grateful you healed yourself for her.

Love, Me

DEAR GRAPPLING FOR PATIENCE

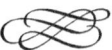

Dear Grappling for Patience,

Oh, by August, most of us have had kids back to school for approximately 2.5 seconds and already bringing home 2.5 viral infections.

I do not know about your kids, but when mine do not feel well, I spend all my energy curating remedies, trying to find what makes them feel better, and I usually turn to my tried-and-true classics.

All the Tylenol administering, heat-pad positioning, chicken-soup making, couch cuddling, movie watching, and popsicle unwrapping to get them to a place of semi-comfort so that I can have some peace and quiet.

Once I think I've covered all the bases, they'll usually cry out: "Mooooooooo-ooooooom. I dooooon't feeeeeeeel gooooooood," on repeat.

That has a tendency to send me over the edge (because I'm

such a patient mom). I have done everything I can possibly think of to make them feel better (and it's never enough), and the only thing I can't help is the time it takes a virus to move through their immune system, so I'll respond back with a not-so-gentle "I know you don't feel good! I don't know what else you want from me!"

Most recently they came back with a just-as-loud "I just want YOU!"

And there it is, friends.

That is all they want... you.

Messy, stressed, impatient, out of ideas but trying her best, giving her all (even if her all is 16%) you.

The next time you feel like you are not doing enough, remember that you ARE enough. Your hands may not be able to cure diseases, but they can certainly soothe some souls.

Love, Me

DEAR LOOKING FOR MORE

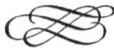

D ear Looking for More,

I have been thinking about something, and it is probably going
to cause a ruckus—but if we have learned anything in this life,
it is that not talking about things does not make them go away.

In fact, it breeds 'em bigger.

So, here is what I have been thinking: what if it is not
enough?

Motherhood, that is.

What if it is everything, but not the only thing?

What if it takes more from us than it gives us?

What if it drains us more than it fills us?

Am I saying that it is not worth it?

No. Because—somehow—beneath the exhausted, ragged,
rundown spirit is a heart so full, it threatens to burst from the
chest.

But what if that is not enough?

What if we have more inside us?

What if we want to be a mom and...?

And a thinker. And a dreamer. And a doer.

Raising kids is more like sowing seeds than growing produce. You plant ideas and values and morals and strength and kindness and love, and you hope it takes. You hope that you have given them the tools to reap the fruits of all that labor.

And sometimes it does, and sometimes it does not. And if we are only moms, then when it does not, that is devastating. But if we are moms and... then maybe a little less devastating.

Therefore, here is what I propose: we can love our kids with everything inside us. We can sacrifice our time, our bodies, and our all to give them everything we got. But sometimes it will not be enough.

In those moments, we have to remember that WE are. We are enough, and it is okay if being a mom is just a part of you.

It is okay to find purpose beyond motherhood.

It is okay to love them fiercely and nurture your passions relentlessly.

It is okay if we give them almost our all and then use that last little bit for ourselves.

Being a mom is everything, but it is not always the only thing, and you know what? I think that dialectical loving is the best kind of living.

Love your kids hard, my friends, but every now and again, love yourself harder.

Love, Me

DEAR WARRIOR

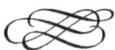

D ear Warrior,

I get skittish when I meet new people and then we become Facebook friends—mostly because I go and friend 'em on Facebook. I suppose that makes me a bit of a masochist, but let us put a pin in that for now.

I also find myself uncomfortable when my coexisting online and real-life friends react to one of my posts. My thoughts become consumed by the realization that they now know.

They know my brain lacks serotonin and that I battle thoughts of self-harm and suicide.

This seems as good a place as any to say that over time—with multiple therapy sessions and just as many medication adjustments—the battle has become a little easier. I can recognize when my depression flares up, and I have the experience to know that it is only temporary even though it feels like an eternity.

Anyway.

I wonder if these fellow Facebookers will still let their kids play with my kids, and if they will tread real light in their interactions with me or write me off completely.

And it makes me realize how strong the stigma around mental illness truly is. So much of "it's all in your head" remains until inner battles are showcased outwardly in the form of addiction, eating disorders, or suicide.

Then we ask why help was not sought sooner. Didn't they know they had an army behind them to walk them through their struggles?

Spoiler alert: they did not.

That is why I write, and that is why I share, and perhaps even overshare. I am not to blame for my mental illness (thank you, trauma and genetics), but I am responsible for my healing and for the years during which I did not want that to be true. It is hard—and quite frankly unfair—to accept responsibility for something I did not cause. But I will be damned if I did not find healing when I accepted both things to be true.

What I want to tell you is that mental illness is not your fault AND you can take control of your healing.

Healing is not linear, and it will probably break your heart while it simultaneously strips you of your defenses. But if you can believe the night is darkest before the dawn, I promise you will find your light.

Keep going, friends; if I have learned anything, it is that you will be glad you did.

Love, Me

DEAR NATURAL BEAUTY WHO DOESN'T SEE IT YET

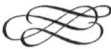

D ear Natural Beauty Who Doesn't See It Yet,

Recently, I told a friend that seeing myself in a photograph has the ability to send me into a ridiculous spiral of self-doubt and loathing.

I have no idea how to position myself in photos, so suffice it to say that my reflection in funhouse mirrors and camera lenses are one and the same.

Which leads us to why I take selfies the way I do. It is a coping mechanism to offset my lack of the photogenic gene. Plus, my self-esteem improves when I can ensure that you know that I know that you know that I am not applying for America's Next Top Model, and I have no idea if that is a relevant comparison anymore because in addition to not being a model, I am also not a spring chicken.

This feels like a good time to say that, believe it or not, I have a point—and fishing for compliments is not it.

A few nights ago, my #4 was going through all the photos stored on my smartphone's memory.

She scrolled on a mission for what seemed like an annoying amount of time and then said, "Mom! You don't have any pictures of yourself."

Not following her point and making my own, I lackadaisically replied with, "That's because I don't need to see myself in pictures."

Y'all, I need you to take a moment and prepare to have your socks knocked off because of what she said next . . .

"But WE do!"

And if there could have been glass that shattered as a symbol of my snapping out of my overly critical, self-deprecating eyes, well, it would have shattered in that moment.

Honestly, I am still reeling from her words.

And now to the point.

It is not breaking news to say we are all our own worst enemies and biggest critics. It hurts less to be the one to say our imperfections out loud before another person recognizes them in us.

But to our kids, we are more than our imperfections, and I kind of want to teach my kids to use their insecurities as their superpowers.

Anyway.

Someday pictures are all my kids will have of the imperfect human that loved them fiercely, so I took a selfie.

And I looked at it like it mattered because it does to them.

Love, Me

DEAR YOU ARE DOING GREAT

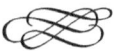

Dear You Are Doing Great,

I do not know if you feel it, but there are not many wins in this parenting gig. I am not blaming them, but the fact that my kids keep score does not help. They keep score for everything.

As in: everything, everything.

Like, I spent twenty-three more seconds saying good night to brother than I did to sister.

Or I asked first-born child about how his day was with more inflection in my voice than I asked second child.

Or I always give youngest kid whatever she wants whenever she wants it and youngest kid never gets punished, but middle child always does.

Or when youngest child asks me how much I love her and I say "infinity," and then she says, "That's it? You could have said a google-o-plex" because apparently that's more than infinity—

and I do not know about you, but I had to Google that because when I took math infinity was the most anything could ever be.

Anyway.

My kids' score-keeping powers are normally used to remind me that I am never fair and that I never say yes. If parenting is not the biggest gaslighting experience of humankind, then I do not know what is.

I think what I'm trying to say is that parenting kids is a mind game that can get you all twisted and turned upside down, and sometimes getting untangled is beyond exhausting; but sometimes your kids surprise you with having each other's backs. This past weekend I watched two of my kids playing soccer for the same team, and the only scores that were kept were when balls went into goals.

There was a moment when my daughter was running herself ragged on the field and my son recognized her subtle signs of exhaustion and called out to the coach with: "My sister needs a break!"

And there was a moment when my son toppled over and under another soccer player, and instead of taking a knee with the rest of the players, my daughter ran over to check on him.

He was fine, by the way.

I live for those moments because they are a reminder that I am not sowing discord among my kids but rather loving them equally in their own unique love language.

All that to say, in those far between moments, the joy of parenting creeps in—and when you let joy creep in, well, that is a win worth soaking in.

Love, Me

DEAR WANTING TO LEAVE

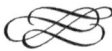

D ear Wanting to Leave,

I started a yoga practice, and let me tell you not a single inch of me was in it. My mind was wandering in all the non-yoga directions, but it did manage to circle back to the same question on repeat, and that question was: "Are we done yet?"

Never have I ever been readier to check an item off my to-do list, but I kept at it because if I have learned anything from my yoga journey it is to show up as you are, and not just notice it but honor it.

So I did.

I wish this was gonna end with an "I feel a million times better," but uh, nope.

Halfway through the practice, a wave of nausea landed front and center, and to be honest it has yet to resolve itself. My chest feels tight-ish, and I am slightly lightheaded as if I might be dehydrated, but I am too worn out to make myself a cup of ice water, and I am too tired to find that lone bottle of trusty peppermint Rolaids that always settles my stomach.

My mind is still wandering, and it is curious as to what is going to happen if I show up on my mat again tomorrow and the next day, and so on and so forth. Even though I don't feel better, I feel curious, and with that curiosity comes hope, which has made pulling my mat out today worth it.

All that to say: showing up isn't always magical. It doesn't always turn your day around. You don't always reap same-day rewards. But sometimes it'll pique your curiosity, and aren't you curious?

What I really want to tell you is: see what happens if you stay.

Love, Me

DEAR DENIAL

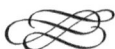

D ear Denial,

Sometimes I think that it is all in my head.

That I don't need to talk about mental health or bring awareness to the internal struggles because if I don't talk about it, then it doesn't exist—and, God, do I wish it didn't exist. But something like this happens:

"Mommy, sometimes I feel claustrophobic and I can't breathe."

In those moments, I am reminded that it is real, and it does happen, and if we act like it doesn't, then we leave our kids without a lifeline when they inevitably feel something that isn't good.

In case you're wondering, I told her that it happens to me too, and we talked about distraction and breathing techniques and she said, "Will coloring help?"

Coloring is one of the coping mechanisms I learned in intensive outpatient therapy, so I said, "That's a great one!"

She went and grabbed her coloring supplies, and she asked me If I wanted to color with her when all I wanted to do was go to bed. But if I can do anything in this life, it'll be to allow my kids to access coping mechanisms as their default, and so I said, "Sure." We colored until she said, "I'm done." I asked her if she felt better, and she said yes.

Mission accomplished.

Mental wellness can be hard to maintain, and at times it may seem futile—but we have little eyes looking to us for guidance in their big feelings, and if nothing else, they're worth fighting for.

Love, Me

DEAR WONDERING IF IT
MATTERS

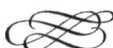

D ear Wondering If It Matters,

I was asked to do a bio for an article, and the request told me to
list the pieces I have written that have gone viral.

Yeah, I left that blank.

I am not the writer or blogger who goes viral. Even when
my work is shared by pages and sites where all their posts go
viral, mine will be the one that doesn't even crack the triple-
digit likes. I actually think the algorithm is out to get me, but
that is a story for another day.

I would be lying if I said that didn't mess with my head
every now and—well, now.

For a while, I had this philosophy that I just needed my
words to be seen by one. One like or one comment or one share
or one view. Just one to feel seen would make the emotional
effort worth it.

But you know what? Sometimes it is not seen by anyone.

Sometimes I put it out there and it goes nowhere. But my soul feels lighter, and in some weird way—even though no one sees it—I feel seen, and don't we all just want to be seen?

What I am trying to tell you is this: if you're doing something that lights a spark inside of you, do it. Don't let the worldly metrics of numbers and reach define its value or worth. Ripple your joy out to your kids and your friends and your partner. They are going to carry that with them, and they are going to do the same. The world needs more ripples and sparks and joy and kindness and community.

You are valuable.

You are worthy.

And if you are the only one you reach, then let that matter.

Love, Me

DEAR LONGING TO BE SEEN

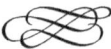

D ear Longing To Be Seen,

At the end of the day, we all just want to be seen. We are longing for it. We are desperate for someone to peer into our souls and tell us that we are worth loving, that we are precious, that we are worth giving it all up for.

I think that's why social media is such a popular concept; it gives us all the chance to be seen. We can put ourselves, our pictures, our ideas, our lives out there, and with the click of a post button we have the chance to be seen by others. But it is all chance.

I think that's what really drew me to Christ—the idea that he sees me exactly as I am and finds me worth loving, and precious, and worth giving it up for. He did give it all up for me and for you and for all of us. And he sees us when no one else does, and not by chance but on purpose.

It doesn't matter if anyone else sees us because we are always seen by him, and I hope that brings you comfort today.

Love, Me

DEAR DEPRESSION HAS ME

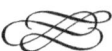

D ear Depression Has Me,

The urgency to leave when depression takes hold can be overwhelming. It threatens to take you deep into a realm of no escape. It is in these moments that self-harm and suicide usually cross my mind. It is a strong pull to follow through—as if my thoughts are all trapped inside and the only thing between me and coveted relief is the constraints of my physical self.

It is what I imagine actual hell to be.

But when the moment passes—and it always, always, always, always passes—I am always, always, always, always grateful that I did not complete either destructive impulse. So if nothing else, I hope this serves as a reminder that your brain will do its best to take you down.

Depression is an actual joy thief, and there is not much you can do when it takes hold except wait for it to pass. Take stock of your unhealthy coping mechanisms and make a mental note when you are not suffering to never implement them. And take the moment to do anything else.

Color.

Meditate.

Run.

Scream.

Declutter.

Clean.

Rearrange furniture.

Walk.

Sit outside.

Turn on a movie or television show you have seen a hundred times and watch it again.

Do anything else. Wait it out. Once it passes, I promise, you'll be glad you did.

Love, Me.

THE END;

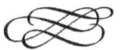

The End;

I have been told a few times:

"*You really put yourself out there in your writing.*"

And I have been ruminating on that the last few days: what do I write about that gives that impression?

I mean, you will never find me talking about specific issues or successes I face in my marriage or in my parenting trials or in my faith tribulations or details about my past trauma or dishing out medical advice to the masses or taking serious selfies because to me THAT is putting myself out there in a way that makes me cringe.

But I do openly share my battles with mental illness, and I can appreciate it is a vulnerable topic for many; once upon a time, it was for me too. But during that time, I was quietly planning my suicide, and that is when I decided there are worse things in life than admitting I live with depression. The worst thing, for me, is living with shame.

One in five people battle a mental illness, and suicide is the tenth leading cause of death, says the National Institute for Mental Health. That just goes to show there are a lot of people waging battles against mental illness but losing the war. Therefore, if my saying that I was once suicidal and I am not now because I spoke up means "putting myself out there," then I guess I do. And I will say it because it may mean you can do so too.

Letting others know they can thrive outside of the darkness is worthwhile because once I realized I was not alone, I believed that I was strong enough to use my voice—and my voice got me help, and that help kept me going.

It just goes to show that everyone has a story they are willing to tell, so share that part of your story freely because your shame will not survive being exposed to the light. By doing so, you will find yourself lighter and brighter and living within a joy you never thought possible, and in the process you might just encourage someone to believe that their story is not over yet.

Do not underestimate the power of your story, warriors; that story could quite literally save a life.

Someone's story saved mine;

And I really hope this one helps save yours.

ACKNOWLEDGMENTS

To Meggan & Lauren: Thank you for believing that if it helps one person, then that is enough. This book literally would not be in the world without your faith in these words and support of these dreams and I am so honored to be linking arms with Starfish Stories Publishing.

To Mary: You're my seester and I don't think I can put into words how much a part of me you are. Thank you for being my sounding board in all the things and life compass in all the ways.

To Amanda: I don't know what I would do without you. Thank you for walking alongside me in this mental health matters journey. I am eternally grateful the soul sister in me found the soul sister in you.

To Andrea: Thank you for believing in my words even when I doubted them. You've been a source of comfort and encouragement since 10th grade and I've always felt seen and accepted by you and I don't think I'll ever be able to fully express my gratitude for your existence.

To Lisa Leshaw: Thank you for popping up in my messages and comments with the most beautiful and kind words. You have restored my faith in humanity- both online and in real life and I adore your spirit.

To Lance: Yes you get a dedication and an acknowledgement because you are my person. You are my rock, my motivational speaker, my confidante, my support system, my co-parent, my love, and my home. Thank you for being in it with me and for ensuring I don't give up on myself.

ABOUT THE AUTHOR

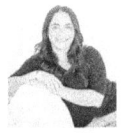

Sara Springer has spent the last two decades supervising the chaos she has created. She is a midwest mom of five and Adult Nurse Practitioner who has battled depression and anxiety for the better part of 30 years. She is now a mental health advocate pursuing her writing dreams. She writes about maintaining mental wellness in parenting, marriage, and online spaces. She is co-founder of the mental health focused non-profit Love Will Foundation, a yoga enthusiast, and a staunch practitioner of sarcasm. Her work has been featured on multiple sites including Her View From Home, Scary Mommy, and The Mighty.

ABOUT STARFISH STORIES PUBLISHING

Starfish Stories Publishing: "Where the woman who reads all the books becomes the woman who writes them."

The Starfish Stories Publishing Company was founded in 2022. Its mission is to create a ripple effect of impact in the world through beautiful storytelling, authentic vulnerability, and inspiring messages of hope and belonging in a world desperate for real connection.

If you have a manuscript you would like us to consider, tap the QR code below and let's chat!

www.ingramcontent.com/pod-product-compliance
Lightning Source LLC
Chambersburg PA
CBHW051004140626
46546CB00016B/192